4/10

¢ 2/14

D0566283

Painkillers

Drugs

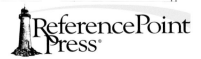

ReferencePoint
Press®

San Diego, CA

Select* books in the Compact Research series include:

Current Issues

Abortion
Animal Experimentation
Biomedical Ethics
Cloning
Conflict in the Middle East
The Death Penalty
Energy Alternatives
Free Speech
Genetic Engineering
Global Warming and
    Climate Change
Gun Control
Illegal Immigration

Islam
Media Violence
National Security
Nuclear Weapons and
    Security
Obesity
School Violence
Stem Cells
Terrorist Attacks
U.S. Border Control
Video Games
World Energy Crisis

Diseases and Disorders

ADHD
Alzheimer's Disease
Anorexia
Autism
Bipolar Disorders
Hepatitis

HPV
Meningitis
Phobias
Sexually Transmitted
    Diseases

Drugs

Alcohol
Antidepressants
Club Drugs
Cocaine and Crack
Hallucinogens
Heroin
Inhalants

Marijuana
Methamphetamine
Nicotine and Tobacco
Performance-Enhancing
    Drugs
Prescription Drugs
Steroids

Energy and the Environment

Biofuels
Deforestation
Hydrogen Power

Solar Power
Wind Power

*For a complete list of titles please visit www.referencepointpress.com.

COMPACT *Research*

Painkillers

Hal Marcovitz

Drugs

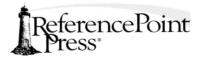

ReferencePoint Press®

San Diego, CA

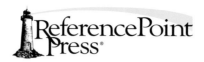

© 2010 ReferencePoint Press, Inc.

For more information, contact:
ReferencePoint Press, Inc.
PO Box 27779
San Diego, CA 92198
www. ReferencePointPress.com

Picture credits:
Cover: iStockphoto.com
AP Images: 17
Science Photo Library: 19
Steve Zmina: 34–36, 48–51, 64–66, 80–83

LIBRARY OF CONGRESS CATALOGING-IN-PUBLICATION DATA

Marcovitz, Hal.
    Painkillers / by Hal Marcovitz.
        p. cm. — (Compact research)
    Includes bibliographical references and index.
    ISBN-13: 978-1-60152-100-2 (hardback)
    ISBN-10: 1-60152-100-6 (hardback)
    1. Analgesics—Popular works. I. Title.
    RM319.M325   2009
    615'.783—dc22

                                                    2009031097

Contents

Foreword

As modern civilization continues to evolve, its ability to create, store, distribute, and access information expands exponentially. The explosion of information from all media continues to increase at a phenomenal rate. By 2020 some experts predict the worldwide information base will double every 73 days. While access to diverse sources of information and perspectives is paramount to any democratic society, information alone cannot help people gain knowledge and understanding. Information must be organized and presented clearly and succinctly in order to be understood. The challenge in the digital age becomes not the creation of information, but how best to sort, organize, enhance, and present information.

ReferencePoint Press developed the *Compact Research* series with this challenge of the information age in mind. More than any other subject area today, researching current issues can yield vast, diverse, and unqualified information that can be intimidating and overwhelming for even the most advanced and motivated researcher. The *Compact Research* series offers a compact, relevant, intelligent, and conveniently organized collection of information covering a variety of current topics ranging from illegal immigration and deforestation to diseases such as anorexia and meningitis.

The series focuses on three types of information: objective single-author narratives, opinion-based primary source quotations, and facts and statistics. The clearly written objective narratives provide context and reliable background information. Primary source quotes are carefully selected and cited, exposing the reader to differing points of view. And facts and statistics sections aid the reader in evaluating perspectives. Presenting these key types of information creates a richer, more balanced learning experience.

For better understanding and convenience, the series enhances information by organizing it into narrower topics and adding design features that make it easy for a reader to identify desired content. For example, in *Compact Research: Illegal Immigration*, a chapter covering the economic impact of illegal immigration has an objective narrative explaining the various ways the economy is impacted, a balanced section of numerous primary source quotes on the topic, followed by facts and full-color illustrations to encourage evaluation of contrasting perspectives.

The ancient Roman philosopher Lucius Annaeus Seneca wrote, "It is quality rather than quantity that matters." More than just a collection of content, the *Compact Research* series is simply committed to creating, finding, organizing, and presenting the most relevant and appropriate amount of information on a current topic in a user-friendly style that invites, intrigues, and fosters understanding.

Painkillers at a Glance

Painkillers Defined

Also known as analgesics and anesthetics, painkillers are drugs that reduce or eliminate pain. Analgesics attack just feelings of pain, and anesthetics eliminate all sensation, causing numbness or inducing the patient to fall asleep.

Two Types of Painkillers

Painkillers fall into two categories: nonprescription and prescription. Nonprescription painkillers include acetaminophen and the nonsteroidal anti-inflammatory drugs, or NSAIDs, which include aspirin, ibuprofen, and naproxen. Prescription painkillers include narcotic drugs known as opioids.

Use of Painkillers

Some 76 million Americans experience pain on a daily basis, including 20 percent who say their pain is chronic, meaning it has continued for three months or more.

How Painkillers Work

Some painkillers reduce inflammation by limiting the body's production of chemicals known as prostaglandins. Other painkillers interact with chemicals in the brain known as neurotransmitters, interrupting messages of pain received by the brain.

Widespread Abuse

Opiate-based painkillers are consumed for their narcotic value, and many people consume nonprescription painkillers in doses above recommended limits under the mistaken belief that larger doses are more effective or act faster.

Severe Consequences

Overuse of acetaminophen has contributed to nearly 500 deaths due to acute liver failure; meanwhile, some 2.1 million teenagers use opiate-based painkillers to get high.

Government Oversight

The federal government keeps a close watch on the development of painkillers and other prescription drugs. It often takes drug companies an investment of more than $1 billion and eight years of clinical trials before painkillers are approved for human consumption.

Many Alternatives

Doctors believe people can ease their pain in many ways without reaching for painkillers. Exercise can help reduce some types of pain. Other therapies, such as massage, acupuncture, and physical therapy, may also ease pain without the use of drugs.

Overview

What Are Painkillers?

Painkillers are drugs that reduce the inflammation that causes pain. They can also block signals of pain that reach the brain or alter the brain's reaction to those signals. Regardless of how they work, painkillers are administered for all manner of injuries and illnesses, helping people overcome the pain they may feel as the result of sudden and traumatic injuries such as broken arms or for constant pain they may experience from chronic ailments such as arthritis or migraine headaches.

Painkillers are also known as analgesics, a term that stems from the Greek words *an* and *algos*, which mean "lacking pain." Pain-reducing drugs can range from mild, nonprescription medications such as aspirin and Tylenol to prescription, opiate-based painkillers such as oxycodone and codeine. Whether they are bought off the shelf at a supermarket or prescribed by a doctor, their intent is the same: to reduce or eliminate the patient's pain.

Some painkillers block all feelings, including pain. These are known as anesthetics, from the Greek words *an* and *aisthisi*, which mean "lacking sensation." The anesthetic Novocain deadens nerves; it is typically injected through a needle by dentists prior to drilling teeth or similar procedures. Novocain is known as a local anesthetic—it affects only a small area of the body. Patients who undergo major surgeries may be put to sleep so that they will not feel the pain of the surgeon's scalpel. These patients have received a drug from a class of painkillers known as general anesthetics. Typically, a general anesthetic is administered through an intravenous tube or in gas form through a mask.

For centuries doctors have sought remedies that would reduce or eliminate pain because for many of their patients, pain is the single most significant symptom of their injuries or illnesses—and it affects the quality of their lives. "Pain is a huge problem, just huge," says Sean Mackey, an assistant professor of pain management at Stanford University School of Medicine in California. "Chronic pain is one of the primary reasons patients go to see the doctor, and the number one reason people are out of work in our society."[1]

Types of Pain

There are two types of pain: acute and chronic. Acute pain often occurs suddenly and without warning: breaking an ankle while sliding into a base while playing baseball will result in immediate and intense pain. In such cases the traumatized part of the body sends an electrical signal to the brain in a process known as nociception. In other words, when a thumb is hit with a hammer, the body is not aware of the pain until the signal travels from the thumb to the brain.

Not all acute pain occurs without warning. A woman approaching childbirth knows the labor and delivery are likely to be painful. A patient suffering from a kidney stone has been told by the doctor that passing the stone will likely result in a painful experience. In all cases, though, acute pain is directly attributable to a specific cause and event. Moreover, acute pain will always go away eventually, sometimes by itself or sometimes with the help of painkillers.

> " For centuries doctors have sought remedies that would reduce or eliminate pain because for many of their patients, pain is the single most significant symptom of their injuries or illnesses. "

Chronic pain, however, is pain that persists over a long period of time—even after the injury that originally caused the pain has healed.

Most doctors define chronic pain as pain that persists for longer than three months.

The cause of chronic pain is often long-term illnesses such as cancer; arthritis, which is an inflammation of the joints; or fibromyalgia, a painful ailment that affects muscles. In many other cases, though, the cause of chronic pain is often a mystery. It is not unusual for patients who have injured their backs to continue feeling aches in their backs for years after their injuries have healed. In this case the feeling of pain has become hardwired into the brain—even after the injury has healed, the brain continues to detect the pain.

> **Most doctors define chronic pain as pain that persists for longer than three months.**

Painkillers are designed to treat pain according to the intensity of the pain and whether the pain is acute or chronic. A mild headache can often be cured with an aspirin. A sports injury such as a sprained ankle may require something stronger, such as ibuprofen. The intense pain of cancer often requires an opiate-based drug. For chronic pain sufferers, doctors may prescribe combinations of drugs over a lengthy period of trial and error until they find the combination that works best for their patients.

Part of Everyday Life

For many people, pain is a part of life: Among them are arthritis patients as well as people who suffer from chronic backaches, cancer patients, and professional athletes whose bodies are constantly under stress. Many people take pain pills several times a week, if not every day. They find the painkillers allow them to pursue normal lives, free of what could be debilitating conditions.

One example of this is Hall of Fame pitcher Nolan Ryan, who lived on pain pills for much of his career in the major leagues. Ryan played in the major leagues for an incredible 27 years. When many pitchers grow older, they often turn to off-speed pitches such as curveballs that take a lot less strength to throw and, therefore, place much less strain on their arms and shoulders. Not Ryan. He spent his entire career as a fastball pitcher; on each pitch, he reached back and threw as hard as he could. Year after year—especially toward the end of his career—Ryan played in pain.

Late in his career, as Ryan prepared to pitch against the Toronto Blue Jays, he was troubled by a sore heel. He took nonprescription painkillers to ease the pain, and went on to pitch a no-hitter. "Once the game started, I didn't notice it,"[2] Ryan said.

A Long History of Fighting Pain

Doctors have searched for centuries for ways to eliminate the pain felt by their patients. Primitive people turned to magic and rituals to drive away pain. They believed pain was caused by evil spirits, and so they put their faith in mystics to drive away the demons causing their pain.

The first doctors believed pain could be eased by drilling holes into the heads of their patients in a procedure known as trepanation. Many archaeologists have unearthed skulls with puncture wounds—evidently, the doctors believed the pain needed a way to get out of the body. The ancient Greek physician Hippocrates, considered the father of modern medicine, advocated trepanning his patients, but Hippocrates also sought out herbal cures. He advised women to chew the bark of a willow tree to deaden the pain they felt during labor and childbirth. Years later chemists distilled the chemical salicylic acid from willow tree bark. Salicylic acid is an active ingredient of aspirin.

> " Many people take pain pills several times a week, if not every day—they find the painkillers allow them to pursue normal lives, free of what could be debilitating conditions. "

Since Hippocrates' time, doctors have tried various other methods of killing pain, often employing herbs but usually relying on other methods as well. In rural America healers concocted a method of pain relief by making a plaster out of hot mustard, then applying it directly to the wound. Under this procedure heat from the plaster was transferred to the ache, which relieved pain. Today doctors call this "counterstimulation"— one source of pain canceling out another.

> **Doctors are not sure how acetaminophen relieves pain, but they suspect it works by expanding the patient's pain threshold—in other words, acetaminophen does not reduce the pain but, instead, helps the patient endure greater amounts of pain.**

As doctors and rural healers tinkered with herbs and mustard plasters, other doctors were learning about the analgesic qualities of opium. The narcotic plant had been cultivated as far back as 3400 B.C.; by the eighteenth century a prosperous opium trade existed between the Far East, where the drug was grown, and customers in Europe. In 1804 the German pharmacist Friedrich Sertürner extracted a painkilling drug from opium. He called it morphine, after Morpheus, the Greek god of dreams.

Morphine was soon employed by military doctors to treat soldiers wounded on the battlefield. The drug was widely used in America during the Civil War; doctors found it enabled them to reduce the pain of their patients while they operated, but many unfortunate soldiers returned home without their limbs or with other battlefield scars and addicted to morphine as well. Following the Civil War, narcotics addiction was known as "soldier's disease."

Modern Advances in Managing Pain

The era of modern painkillers commenced in 1893 when a German chemist, Felix Hoffman, found a way to make salicylic acid digestible. He buffered the acid by adding salt and the chemical acetyl chloride to create acetylsalicylic acid. Doctors had known for centuries that salicylic acid possessed analgesic qualities, but most people could not take the drug because it caused upset stomachs. Hoffman pursued his research because his father suffered from a painful condition of the joints that was probably arthritis. It is believed Hoffman may have actually come across a formula for buffering salicylic acid discovered 40 years before by a French chemist, Charles-Frédéric Gerhardt. Nevertheless, Hoffman is given credit for the discovery, and the German company where he worked, Bayer, soon became the world's largest manufacturer of the new drug, which was called aspirin. Bayer created the name for the drug by combining the letter *a*, which stands for acetylsalicylic, with the word *spir*, taken from the Latin name for the herb meadowsweet, *Spiraea ulmaria*, which provided the salicylic acid for the formula.

During the twentieth century many additional advances in the development of painkillers took place. Acetaminophen gained widespread use in the 1950s: The first product under the name Tylenol was introduced by its manufacturer, McNeil Laboratories, in 1955. In 1969 British doctors first employed ibuprofen as a painkilling drug for their arthritis patients. In the 1980s the use of opiate-based drugs was widely employed for cancer patients, whose doctors believed they should not have to suffer as they went through the severe pain common in the disease. This was the era in which the opiate oxycodone was first widely used as a painkiller. The two most widely used brand-name drugs composed of oxycodone are OxyContin and Percocet. Other well-known opiate-based painkillers are propoxyphene, sold under the brand name Darvocet, and hydrocodone, available under the brand name Vicodin. Oxycodone and other opiate-based painkillers are available only by prescription and are usually administered to patients whose pain is unceasing and relentless.

> **Essentially, opiates fool the brain into believing there is no pain.**

How Do Painkillers Affect the Body?

Aspirin reduces pain by inhibiting the production of prostaglandins, which are chemicals that help the blood clot. In addition, prostaglandins make nerve endings more sensitive to pain. Aspirin also possesses anti-inflammatory properties; in other words, it reduces swelling, which is a painful condition that occurs following a sprain or similar injury.

Other common nonprescription anti-inflammatory drugs include ibuprofen, which is found in Advil and Motrin, and naproxen, the active ingredient of Aleve. Like aspirin, they inhibit the production of prostaglandins. Aspirin, ibuprofen, and naproxen are known as nonsteroidal anti-inflammatory drugs, or NSAIDs. As the name indicates, NSAIDs do not include steroids, which are part of a wide-ranging class of drugs known for their abuse among athletes who use them to build muscle mass. However, steroids also have anti-inflammatory properties and, therefore, can be employed as painkillers. However, steroids are not found in nonprescription analgesics.

> " In the weeks following Michael Jackson's death, reports surfaced that the singer had endured a long-term addiction to prescription painkillers. "

Another nonprescription pain reliever is acetaminophen. Doctors are not sure how acetaminophen relieves pain, but they suspect it works by expanding the patient's pain threshold—in other words, acetaminophen does not reduce the pain but instead helps the patient endure greater amounts of pain.

Opiates such as codeine and oxycodone go directly to the brain, interacting with the neurotransmitters, the chemicals manufactured by the brain that control physical and mental functions. Essentially, opiates fool the brain into believing there is no pain. "Opiates . . . are highly effective medications when properly used for the management of acute pain," say authors and addiction experts Jeff Jay and Jerry A. Boriskin. "Opiates are often prescribed following surgery because their ability to block pain helps patients get out of bed sooner, which contributes to healing."[3]

What Are the Dangers of Painkillers?

Addiction to opiate-based painkillers is common. Most people know Paula Abdul as a former judge on *American Idol*. Since the age of 17, when she suffered an injury as a cheerleader, Abdul has lived with pain. Over the years she has also suffered a broken leg while rehearsing and was injured in a car accident and later a small airplane crash. Along the way she became addicted to painkillers.

Finally, she went through drug rehab to kick her addiction. As she learned, kicking an addiction to opiate-based painkillers is no different than kicking an addiction to heroin or cocaine. Her body had to go through the agonies of withdrawal as she weaned herself off the narcotic.

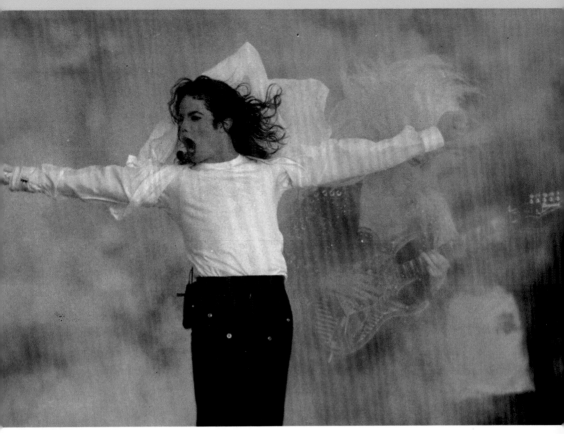

In a memorable performance, pop star Michael Jackson sings and dances during the 1993 Super Bowl halftime show. In the weeks after Jackson's death in June 2009, reports surfaced that the singer had a long-term addiction to prescription painkillers.

"It's the worst thing," she says. "I was freezing cold, then sweating hot, then chattering and in so much pain. It was excruciating, but at my very core I did not like existing the way I had been."[4]

Among other celebrities who have admitted to having painkiller addictions are Cindy McCain, wife of 2008 presidential candidate John McCain; radio talk show host Rush Limbaugh; quarterbacks Brett Favre and Ryan Leaf; and Nicole Richie, Winona Ryder, Matthew Perry, Kelly and Jack Osbourne, Jamie Lee Curtis, Eminem, Courtney Love, and Charlie Sheen.

In 2009 pop star Michael Jackson was found dead in his home at the age of 50. In the weeks following Jackson's death, reports surfaced that the singer had endured a long-term addiction to prescription painkillers.

After an investigation, authorities determined that Jackson died after a doctor administered an overdose of the anesthetic propofol. The drug is employed by anesthesiologists to put people to sleep before surgeries, but Jackson had been using it to combat insomnia.

How Does the Government Regulate Painkillers?

Before painkillers are sold over the counter or by prescription, they must receive the approval of the U.S. Food and Drug Administration (FDA). Typically, it takes drug manufacturers several years to win FDA approval. The agency requires extensive tests and trials of painkillers, as well as all other drugs, before it approves them for use in America.

Even after painkillers have been on the market for several years, the government constantly reviews their effectiveness and safety. In 2009 an FDA advisory panel reviewed the safety of acetaminophen and found the drug contributes to liver failure. The panel cited statistics showing that during the 1990s, overuse of acetaminophen contributed to 56,000 emergency room visits, 26,000 hospitalizations, and 458 deaths. Specifically, the advisory panel found that acetaminophen contributes to liver damage.

Acetaminophen is by no means an obscure drug—it is the active ingredient in Tylenol, one of the most familiar painkillers available without a prescription. According to the FDA, Americans consume 28 billion doses of acetaminophen a year.

> **Many doctors are convinced that if the brain does not know about pain, the pain will cease.**

Clearly, though, the FDA panel is concerned that Americans consume too much acetaminophen. According to the instructions printed on labels for Extra Strength Tylenol, the maximum daily consumption should not exceed 4,000 milligrams, or 8 tablets. The FDA panel recommended that the maximum daily dose be reduced to 2,600 milligrams. The FDA is not compelled to accept the advisory panel's recommendations; nevertheless, members of the group said they are confident the agency would follow their advice. "I think this is the one place where we can engineer safety," said Judith

Kramer, an advisory panel member and associate professor of medicine at Duke University Medical Center in North Carolina. "We're here because there are inadvertent overdoses that are fatal, and this is our one opportunity to have a big impact."[5]

Are There Alternatives to Painkillers?

Science has developed some new ways to eliminate pain without resorting to drugs. Ultrasound is a familiar technique that has been used for

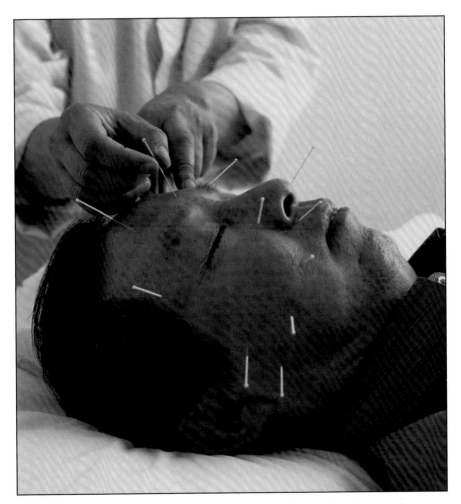

An acupuncturist inserts needles into a patient's skin. Placed at specific points of the body, the needles are thought to disrupt the flow of pain. Some Western experts also believe that the needles stimulate the release of endorphins, which are the body's natural painkillers.

years to create images of babies in the womb, but doctors have also found it is effective for loosening sore tissue that causes pain. The sound waves create heat, which improves blood flow and reduces swelling, making sore muscles and joints more responsive to stretching exercises that can help alleviate pain.

TENS is another alternative to drug therapy. TENS stands for transcutaneous electrical nerve stimulation. A TENS pad is placed against an area of the body that is in pain; the pad then transmits a mild electrical shock that sends a stimulating signal to the brain, scrambling the signals of pain that are being emitted by the achy body part. Patients say TENS provides a pleasing, prickly feeling.

For more serious cases involving back pain, an electrode can be inserted into the spine to provide direct electrical stimulation. This procedure is known as intradiscal electrothermal therapy. In many severe cases of back pain, the aches are often caused by damaged intervertebral discs, which act as cushions for the bones in the spine. Intradiscal electrothermal therapy uses the electrical charge to create heat and deaden the nerve endings in the discs, thus eliminating the pain.

The Brain Is the Source

Many doctors are convinced that if the brain does not know about pain, the pain will cease. Some of the most cutting-edge research in pain management is being performed on the brain, providing direct electrical stimulation to parts of the brain that detect pain.

The technique is known as deep brain stimulation. Doctors believe they can find the specific areas of the brain that respond to the painful impulses transmitted by the rest of the body. Doctors suspect that the part of the brain known as the thalamus may be the location for many pain receptors. By inserting an electrode directly into the thalamus and providing a mild electrical shock, doctors believe that very severe pain can be made to go away.

The thalamus is located deep inside the brain, meaning that a patient would have to undergo significant surgery in order to participate in the stimulation. The electrode remains embedded permanently in the thalamus, its power provided by batteries. Constant electrical pulses are transmitted into the brain, interrupting the painful sensations emitted elsewhere in the body. Deep brain stimulation has been used on about

700 patients, with many reporting a 100 percent success rate in eliminating their pain.

Deep brain stimulation as well as other techniques that can disperse pain without the need for drugs are still in the experimental phases and are not likely to be available to most people for many years. For the near future, it would seem that most pain sufferers will continue reaching for their pain pills for as long as they feel pain.

How Do Painkillers Affect the Body?

"No medals are awarded for suffering. One of the dumbest things I ever did was refuse painkillers when I had my colon out back in 1984. I was 27 and had been raised in a stoic rural culture in which I was taught that only lightweights and losers took pain pills."

—*New York Times* editor and cancer survivor Dana Jennings.

What Is Pain?

It is not easy to define pain, since the threshold of pain is different for everybody: What is painful for one person may not be painful for somebody else. A professional boxer, for example, is able to withstand constant blows to the head and other physical punishments that most other people would find unbearable.

Other athletes also possess high thresholds of pain. National Football League (NFL) quarterback Donovan McNabb once broke his ankle early in a game, refused to come out of the game, and went on to throw four touchdown passes while leading his team to victory. "For someone able to do something like that . . . they have a very high pain tolerance," says Jeff Anderson, director of sports medicine at the University of Connecticut. "And that really varies, person to person. Certain people feel pain differently than others."[6] Most people who break their ankles would find it difficult to put the slightest weight on their broken bones. To them the idea of playing an entire professional football game on such a serious injury would be unthinkable.

The International Association for the Study of Pain, which is composed of physicians who treat pain, has defined pain as "an unpleasant sensory and emotional experience associated with actual or potential tissue damage." The organization adds, though, that "pain is always subjective. Each individual learns the application of the word through experiences related to injury in early life."[7] Essentially, individuals develop their own ideas about pain and how much they can endure before they require relief. That is why professional boxers or football players, who may endure painful blows for years, are able to perform at top levels even though they have sustained serious injuries, while others would become severely debilitated should they suffer similar injuries.

"A Hidden Disease"

Pain impedes the joy of life, forcing patients to remain apart from others. Pain makes people miss school and work and keeps them from living full lives. Says Raymond Gaeta, associate professor of anesthesia at Stanford University Hospital and School of Medicine, "Pain has been a hidden disease; it has not received as much attention as other diseases, but now there's a growing recognition that pain really is not just the sensation we have—it's something that interferes with every one of us, with life."[8]

Some 76 million people experience pain on a daily basis, with more than half of adults over the age of 20 reporting that their pain is chronic, meaning it has lasted for at least 3 months. Many patients suffer from well-known diseases such as cancer and AIDS, but many also suffer from obscure diseases such as reflex sympathetic dystrophy, a mysterious ailment that struck ballet student Cynthia Toussaint as she was stretching at the barre. Toussaint

> " A professional boxer . . . is able to withstand constant blows to the head and other physical punishments that most other people would find unbearable. "

felt a pain shoot down her leg and at first thought it was nothing more than a muscle pull. That was in 1983. Within a few weeks Toussaint was confined to her bed as the pain persisted. Since then she has spent most of her life in a wheelchair. "It feels like I've been doused with gasoline and lit on fire,"[9] she says.

How Does the Body React to an Injury?

When the body is injured it summons its own defensive mechanisms. When an ankle is sprained—meaning the ligaments in the ankle tear or are stretched too far—the condition usually results in swelling, also known as inflammation. Swelling occurs because tiny blood vessels have been ruptured. Also, the body sends blood and various chemicals, known as circulating immune complexes, to the injury so the healing process can begin. These chemicals and the extra blood also contribute to swelling. The inflammation causes pain because the blood and chemicals press against the nerve endings in the injured part of the body.

Certainly, pain is unpleasant, but it is not necessarily a bad reaction to an injury. Pain can be regarded as a good signal, alerting the patient to trouble. "When something goes wrong, your body has ways of telling you," says Darin Workman, a Texas-based chiropractic physician. "The sign that we most commonly notice is pain. . . . Pain is our body's fire alarm to warn us that problems exist."[10]

Most inflammation goes away after a few hours or few days, but some inflammation is chronic—the inflammation caused by arthritis is constant and difficult to treat. Long-lasting inflammation can be destructive and cause permanent disability to joints and muscles as well as constant pain.

The Mildest Painkillers

One way to kill pain is to reduce the flow of the pain-causing chemicals that are rushing to the location of the inflammation. Aspirin, ibuprofen, and naproxen accomplish this goal by inhibiting the body's release of a chemical known as cyclooxygenase, or COX. COX helps convert fatty acids found in cell walls into prostaglandins. The prostaglandins are among the chemicals released by the body in response to an injury. These drugs are NSAIDs—anti-inflammatory painkillers that are available over the counter. They can be effective for mild headaches, joint pain, menstrual cramps, sore backs, and other conditions that are not considered chronic.

Acetaminophen also blocks the release of COX but not as effectively as aspirin, ibuprofen, and naproxen. Still, it is an effective painkiller for headaches and minor pain. Doctors believe it works by expanding the patient's pain threshold, although they are not sure exactly how it does this.

In 1988 doctors discovered that there are two types of COX found in the body: COX-1 and COX-2. COX-1 is found throughout the body and has many functions, including a role in the production of the natural mucus lining of the stomach. COX-2, however, is found only in inflamed tissue. Aspirin, ibuprofen, and naproxen inhibit COX-1 and COX-2. Therefore, some bad side effects could surface by using painkillers that block COX-1, such as upset stomachs. Acetaminophen blocks COX-2 only. Therefore, acetaminophen is considered to be gentler on the stomach than aspirin and the other NSAIDs.

> " Pain is unpleasant, but it is not necessarily a bad reaction to an injury. Pain can be regarded as a good signal, alerting the patient to trouble. "

Painkillers by Prescription

Another way of reducing pain is to interrupt the pain impulse in the brain—essentially, to fool the brain into believing the injury is not painful. For pain that is chronic and intense—such as the pain that may be suffered by a cancer patient—doctors may prescribe opiate-based painkillers. These painkillers include drugs such as codeine (Tylenol 3), hydrocodone (Vicodin), oxycodone (OxyContin and Percocet), and propoxyphene (Darvocet). They are all narcotic-based drugs, known as opioids, that react by enhancing or altering the flow of chemicals known as neurotransmitters, thereby blocking transmissions of pain.

Neurotransmitters are chemicals that carry messages from brain cell to brain cell. Neurotransmitters relay instructions, telling the hand when to lift a fork, the heart when to beat, or the body when to grow tired and seek sleep. Neurotransmitters also control feelings of pleasure and pain.

Drugs can have an enormous effect on neurotransmitters, altering how they work—this is how illegal drugs such as heroin and cocaine provide the narcotic highs experienced by users.

Painkillers target neurotransmitters that directly affect the sensations of pain. One of those neurotransmitters is serotonin, which controls sensory experiences, sleep, and mood. Opioids enhance the flow of serotonin, which helps reduce pain. Another neurotransmitter affected by opioids is norepinephrine, which controls blood pressure and pulse rate. By speeding up pulse rate and increasing blood pressure, the natural healing powers of the blood are enhanced, helping to reduce pain.

> **Another way of reducing pain is to interrupt the pain impulse in the brain—essentially, to fool the brain into believing the injury is not painful.**

Opioids also enhance the effectiveness of natural chemicals known as endorphins. These are chemicals produced by the body during periods of stress, including times when the body is in pain. Long-distance runners often experience what they refer to as the "runner's high," which occurs when they are at the point of exhaustion and pain. Suddenly, the exhaustion and pain go away and they are able to continue the race—this feeling occurs at the moment when their endorphins get a natural kick-start. People who suffer from chronic pain also find relief through the release of their endorphins, only in their cases the endorphins are released with the help of painkilling drugs. "Prescription pain medications are essentially all related by their common effect on the body's endorphin system,"[11] says Drew Pinsky, a Pasadena, California, physician and medical writer.

Making Migraines Go Away

People who suffer from migraine headaches describe the pain as intense and unpredictable. Terri Burchfield, a 41-year-old resident of McLean, Virginia, has been stricken with migraines that are so bad she has been forced to find relief in hospital emergency rooms. "I was doubled over in pain," Burchfield recalls of a recent migraine attack. "The head pain was so severe, it was emanating throughout my entire body. I've never had pain that even comes close."[12]

The pain of migraines often does not respond to nonprescription anti-inflammatory drugs; moreover, doctors do not feel comfortable prescribing opioids to migraine patients who are otherwise healthy individuals. Migraines are believed to have many causes—diet, stress, even the weather.

Many people who suffer from migraines are treated with a class of prescription drugs known as triptans, which get their name from the active ingredient, the chemical tryptamine. Triptans enhance the flow of serotonin without the use of opiates. Also, triptans constrict the size of the blood vessels in the brain; therefore, they have anti-inflammatory effects.

What Is Anesthesia?

Most everyone who has spent time in a dentist's chair has experienced the numbing effects of Novocain. When injected, the local anesthetic temporarily deadens nerves so that minor surgeries, such as filling cavities or extracting teeth, can be performed pain free. Novocain works by changing the chemistry of the membranes that act as a gateway for sodium and potassium to pass in and out of nerve cells. This exchange of sodium and potassium enables the nerve cells to feel impulses—in the case of a visit to the dentist, the stabbing pain of a high-speed drill.

Novocain slows the transfer of sodium, which prevents transmission of the physical impulse. Since it is an anesthetic, it kills all sensation, not just pain. Novocain, which is injected with a needle, acts within two to five minutes and lasts for an hour or more, depending on how much the dentist uses.

> People who suffer from chronic pain also find relief through the release of their endorphins, only in their cases the endorphins are released with the help of painkilling drugs.

Novocain and similar drugs, such as procaine and lidocaine, are also used for other medical procedures, including some spinal surgeries. Local anesthesia is also employed during childbirth—many women receive injections of local anesthetics in their spines in procedures known as epidurals. The anesthetic is injected into a soft part of the spinal column, deadening sensations in the pelvic area and allowing the women to give birth without pain.

> "Novocain, which is injected with a needle, acts within two to five minutes and lasts for an hour or more, depending on how much the dentist uses."

General anesthesia has a long history of use that dates back to 1845, when dentists first administered nitrous oxide to their patients. The gas is a weak general anesthesia. It does not put patients to sleep, but rather makes them slightly intoxicated—it is used to sedate patients who fear the dentist's chair.

Today general anesthesia is used to put patients to sleep during surgeries. It is administered in gas form through face masks or liquid form through intravenous tubes by specialists known as anesthesiologists. To put a patient to sleep, the physician will give the patient a dose of drugs known as benzodiazepines, which work by interacting with neurotransmitters that induce sleep. It is also likely that the anesthesiologist will provide the patient with a so-called induction drug, which will speed up the effect of the benzodiazepine. Finally, the anesthesiologist will probably also inject the patient with an opiate-based painkiller so that the patient will remain pain free once he or she wakes up after the surgery.

Managing Chronic Pain

For many patients, painkilling pills are not enough to manage their pain. Some patients undergo patient-controlled analgesia, in which they are hooked to an intravenous line that feeds a constant stream of painkilling drugs into their bodies; the patients themselves control the pumps, releasing the medication as needed. In many cases people who are recovering from extensive surgeries are provided with such pumps. Other patients make regular visits to their doctors to receive trigger point injections. These are injections of painkilling drugs, usually local anesthetics, that go right to the trouble points.

Clearly, there is a wide variety of painkilling drugs, each affecting the body in different ways. Some patients find they need just an occasional aspirin to make their headaches go away. Others who are recovering from significant surgeries must have access to a constant stream of drugs in order for them to endure their long and otherwise painful recoveries. People like Cynthia Toussaint never escape their pain; they are forced to endure life in constant pain. And then there are people like Donovan McNabb who can break an ankle on the third play from scrimmage and then go on to have a career day, throwing four touchdown passes without showing the slightest wince.

Primary Source Quotes*

How Do Painkillers Affect the Body?

"In the hospital, the morphine drip is a mighty stream. If you need it, don't be afraid, just wade in."

—Dana Jennings, "Post-Op Strategies: Painkillers, to Start," *New York Times*, January 27, 2009.

Jennings is a cancer patient and an editor at the *New York Times*.

"Painkillers are not real solutions . . . let alone cures; they merely mask the pain. Giving a painkiller to relieve . . . pain is a little like taking the battery out of a smoke alarm because the noise is too loud."

—Todd Sinett and Sheldon Sinett, *The Truth About Back Pain*. New York: Perigee, 2008.

Todd Sinett and Sheldon Sinett are New York City–based chiropractic physicians and the authors of the book *The Truth About Back Pain*.

* Editor's Note: While the definition of a primary source can be narrowly or broadly defined, for the purposes of Compact Research, a primary source consists of: 1) results of original research presented by an organization or researcher; 2) eyewitness accounts of events, personal experience, or work experience; 3) first-person editorials offering pundits' opinions; 4) government officials presenting political plans and/or policies; 5) representatives of organizations presenting testimony or policy.

❝ Pain is that experience we associate with actual or potential tissue damage. It is unquestionably a sensation in a part or parts of the body, but it is also always unpleasant and therefore also an emotional experience. ❞

—International Association for the Study of Pain, "Pain Terminology," November 29, 2007. www.iasp-pain.org.

The International Association for the Study of Pain is the professional association of physicians who specialize in treating pain.

❝ Pain is a complex process, and the pain signal can be magnified, minimized, and reinterpreted by a person's experiences, both past and present. ❞

—Margaret A. Caudill, *Managing Pain Before It Manages You*. New York: Guilford, 2009.

Caudill is a physician who specializes in pain management and is an instructor in anesthesiology at Dartmouth Hitchcock Medical Center in Lebanon, New Hampshire.

❝ The physician has an obligation to relieve a patient's pain and suffering. Despite good intentions and genuine concern for patients' comfort on the part of physicians, repeated evaluations of the state of pain therapy over the past 20 years suggest that many patients do not receive adequate pain relief. ❞

—American Medical Association Council on Scientific Affairs, "Aspects of Pain Management in Adults," July 1, 2009. www.ama-assn.org.

The American Medical Association is a professional organization representing nearly 250,000 doctors.

❝ Pain management as a human right is a moral imperative that will help medicine return to its humanist roots. Acknowledging this right is a crucial step in reversing the public health crisis of undertreated pain. ❞

—Scott M. Fishman, "Recognizing Pain Management as a Human Right: A First Step," *Anesthesia & Analgesia*, July 2007.

Fishman is the chief of pain management and a professor of anesthesiology at the University of California–Davis.

❝I became so consumed with my pain that all of my energies were focused on the pain, how to rid my body of unrelenting pain, and getting back to life the way it was before pain. . . . It made no sense to me that with all the modern miracles in medicine there was no way to relieve my pain.❞

—Penny Cowan, "Driving with Four Flat Tires," *American Chronic Pain Association Chronicle*, September 2008.

Cowan is the executive director of the American Chronic Pain Association.

❝It's easy to feel overwhelmed when you live with chronic pain. . . . It's especially frustrating when family, friends, even doctors and nurses tell you that you should be feeling better, you're not trying hard enough, you're addicted to pain pills or that you're just a complainer.❞

—Rebecca Rengo, "How to Live Well with Chronic Pain," 2006. www.beyondchronicpain.com.

Rengo is a social worker, the president of the Missouri Pain Initiative, and the author of the book *Beyond Chronic Pain*.

How Do Painkillers Affect the Body?

- More than **50 percent** of women who give birth elect to ease the pain of childbirth through epidural anesthesia.

- About **50 percent** of all American dentists use nitrous oxide to sedate their patients.

- The *Journal of Pain* reports that **a third** of people who are in pain say their pain is disabling, which is defined as severe and having a high impact on the quality of their lives.

- About **80 percent** of Americans will suffer from back pain at least once in their lives.

- A study by Harvard University found that **93 percent** of migraine patients who take triptans report pain relief within 20 minutes of the onset of their headaches.

- Although opiate-based painkillers are typically prescribed to cancer patients, as many as **75 percent** of cancer patients who die experience moderate to severe pain during their final days.

- **One in five** Americans takes a nonprescription painkiller at least once a week.

- Americans consume more than **50 million** aspirin tablets a day, or roughly more than **18 billion** per year.

Relieving Pain with Prescription Painkillers

Americans have increasingly found relief from pain with the help of prescription painkillers. The U.S. Agency for Healthcare Research and Quality reports that American doctors wrote more than 230 million prescriptions for painkillers in 2006—about 40 percent more than they wrote in 1996.

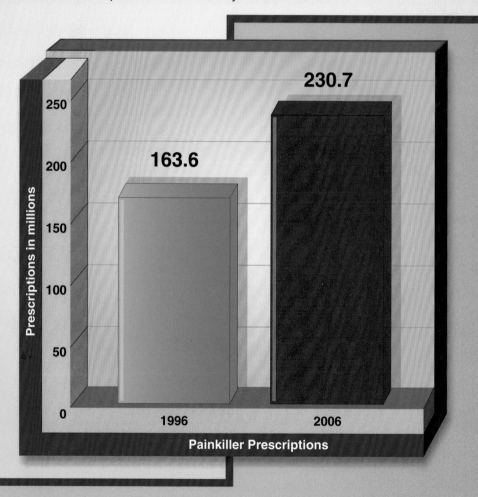

Source: Marie N. Stagnitti, "Trends in Outpatient Prescription Analgesics Utilization and Expenditures for the U.S. Civilian Noninstitutional Population, 1996 and 2006," U.S. Agency for Healthcare Research and Quality, February 2009. www.meps.ahrq.gov.

- According to the U.S. Food and Drug Administration, acetaminophen is an ingredient in more than **600 prescription and over-the-counter medications**.

Many Americans Live with Pain

Large numbers of Americans suffer from pain, and they are turning to painkillers for relief as never before. Between 1997 and 2005, sales of 5 major painkillers rose nearly 90 percent, according to a 2007 Associated Press analysis of Drug Enforcement Administration statistics. More than 25 percent of all adults suffer from low back pain; knee pain and headaches also plague many Americans over the age of 18, according to the Centers for Disease Control and Prevention.

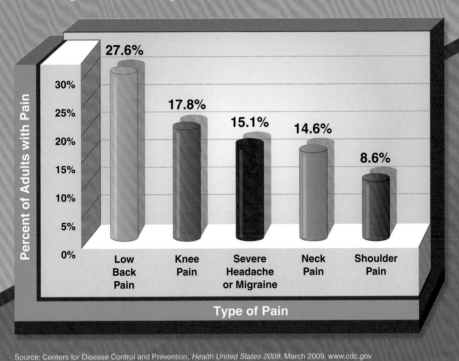

Source: Centers for Disease Control and Prevention, *Health United States 2008*, March 2009. www.cdc.gov.

- Between 1996 and 2006 the U.S. Food and Drug Administration approved the use of **10 drugs** to treat migraine headache pain.

- Americans consume more than **100 tons** (90.7 metric tons) a year of **opiate-based painkillers** such as codeine, morphine, oxycodone, and hydrocodone, according to the U.S. Drug Enforcement Administration.

How Long Does Pain Last?

Chronic pain is regarded as pain that lasts 3 months or longer, but many American adults endure pain that lasts longer than that. In fact, according to the American Pain Foundation, 14 percent of people over the age of 20 say their pain lasts up to a year while 42 percent say they have endured pain for a year or more. To treat their chronic conditions, many Americans turn to drugs that relieve pain.

Duration of Pain

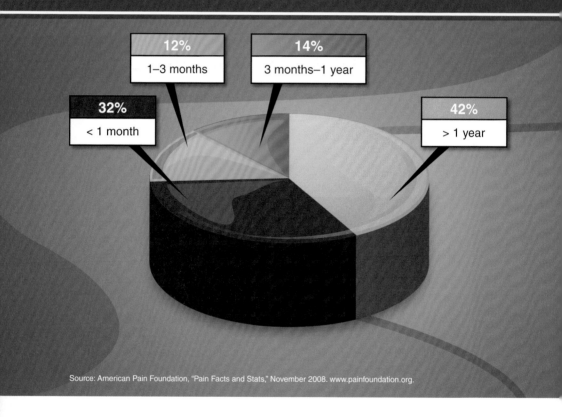

12%
1–3 months

14%
3 months–1 year

32%
< 1 month

42%
> 1 year

Source: American Pain Foundation, "Pain Facts and Stats," November 2008. www.painfoundation.org.

- **One in four** American households includes at least one person who suffers from migraine headaches; three out of four migraine sufferers are women.

What Are the Dangers of Painkillers?

“When prescription drugs are abused in the same way as illegal street drugs, they're every bit as addictive and every bit as deadly.”

—Steve Pasierb, president of the Partnership for a Drug-Free America.

Desperate and Devious

Sam Rayburn joined the Philadelphia Eagles in 2003 and soon established himself as one of the team's toughest young players. It seemed as though Rayburn was on the brink of a long and lucrative career as a defensive lineman in the NFL, but then he suffered through a series of injuries to his knees, elbow, and spine that ended his career after just four seasons. Even though his career in the NFL was over, the pain caused by his injuries persisted. To deal with the pain, Rayburn consumed prescription painkillers. Soon he was addicted to the opiate-based substances. "You double the dosage that you normally take, and that leads to a higher tolerance, and then you need more to get the same effect," says Rayburn. "Eventually, it kind of snowballs out of control. The next thing you know, you're taking 100 a day. And you really don't know how you got there."[13]

No doctor would write prescriptions for Rayburn to obtain the drugs he needed to feed his habit, so he turned to desperate and devious measures that included stealing prescription pads, forging the scrips for

> **To deal with the pain, Rayburn consumed prescription painkillers. Soon he was addicted to the opiate-based substances.**

Percocet and Lortab, a hydrocodone painkiller, and sending teenagers into pharmacies to have them filled. Police finally caught up with Rayburn in 2009. He was arrested and charged with a number of drug offenses.

Under the authority of the court, Rayburn did find help—he went through a rehabilitation program and managed to kick his addiction to prescription painkillers. Of his former addiction, Rayburn says: "It gets to the point where you don't need them for the pain, you need them just to function. You need them to eat, to sleep, to get up—to do anything at all. You can't even watch TV without taking pills because that's the first thing on your mind."[14]

What Is Pharming?

The opiate content of prescription painkillers such as Percocet, Vicodin, and OxyContin has proved to be irresistible to many drug abusers, particularly young drug abusers. Many teenagers raid the medicine cabinets at home, taking the prescription pain-relieving drugs obtained by their parents. This is known as "pharming." According to the White House Office of National Drug Control Policy, each year 2.1 million people between the ages of 12 and 17 use prescription painkillers to get high. In fact, the only drug that young people abuse more than prescription painkillers is marijuana, but even that trend may be changing. Among teens, the number of first-time abusers of prescription drugs now exceeds the number of first-time users of marijuana.

This abuse of prescription painkillers among teens can be particularly dangerous. When doctors prescribe opiate-based painkillers, they usually provide specific instructions on how they are to be taken. One of the most common instructions that accompanies a prescription for painkillers is to avoid consumption of alcohol while taking the painkiller. Narcotic painkillers and alcohol are both depressants—meaning they both depress, or slow, the functions of the body's vital organs. When mixed they can multiply each other's effects—slowing the heart rate or respiratory function to dangerously low, even fatal, levels.

Young drug abusers often do not realize the consequences of mixing alcohol with an opiate-based painkiller. Says a 2008 report by the Office of National Drug Control Policy, "Teens who abuse prescription or over-the-counter drugs may be abusing other substances as well. Sometimes they abuse prescription and over-the-counter drugs together with alcohol or other drugs, which can lead to dangerous consequences, including death."[15]

The Arrival of Hillbilly Heroin

OxyContin was regarded as a breakthrough painkiller because it was designed to release its main ingredient, oxycodone, over the course of several hours. That meant a cancer patient or other person suffering from intense and chronic pain need only take one or two doses a day, making it likely that the effects of the painkiller would remain constant.

However, drug abusers soon found that if they crushed the pill with their teeth, they could get the entire narcotic hit at once. Many abusers describe the high as similar to the narcotic effect of heroin. OxyContin has gained the nickname "hillbilly heroin" because of its widespread use in rural communities, but in reality, abuse of the drug is common in cities and suburbs as well.

According to the U.S. Drug Enforcement Administration, the most common way of obtaining OxyContin is by "doctor shopping"—a drug dealer makes appointments to see multiple doctors across town, then convinces or cons those doctors into writing prescriptions for OxyContin. The drug dealers then get the prescriptions filled at a number of pharmacies. Now possessing several bottles containing dozens or even hundreds of tablets, the dealers hit the streets, where they sell the pills one by one to abusers—getting as much as $25 or $40 per pill.

> **Many teenagers raid the medicine cabinets at home, taking the prescription pain-relieving drugs obtained by their parents.**

Other drug dealers who are not as savvy or otherwise cannot con a doctor into writing a prescription have much more direct methods of obtaining OxyContin: Burglaries and armed robberies of pharmacies are common occurrences in America. At one recent robbery at a pharmacy in Lillington, North Carolina, two armed robbers entered the store at closing time, drew guns, and stole only quantities of OxyContin and Percocet. The drugs had a retail value of $10,000, but officials believed the two robbers could get many times that amount for the drugs as they sold them pill by pill. "He said he wanted only OxyContin," pharmacy worker Lisa Ledford said of one of the robbers. "He told us the robbery was for real and said if we did what he said nobody would get hurt."[16]

Abuse of Nonprescription Painkillers

Nonprescription painkillers do not offer a narcotic high, but they are still abused—a trend that led the advisory panel of the Food and Drug Administration to recommend reducing the maximum dosage of products containing acetaminophen. Some people who experience acute pain for what are usually minor injuries may overdose on the over-the-counter products, swallowing many times the recommended dosage and hoping for quick and immediate relief from their pain.

> **Some people who experience acute pain for what are usually minor injuries may overdose on the over-the-counter products, swallowing many times the recommended dosage and hoping for quick and immediate relief from their pain.**

One survey conducted by the National Consumers League found that 44 percent of people who take nonprescription painkillers admit to exceeding the recommended dosages spelled out on the labels. Says Linda Golodner, president of the National Consumers League: "Our survey results are disheartening, but they reflect what we suspected about the behavior of those in great discomfort. Too often, consumers just want the pain to go away, so they take more medicine than the label instructs, and they don't talk to their doctor about the possible risks."[17]

What many people do not realize, however, is that taking doses that are larger than the maximum recommended amount provides just minimal increases in the analgesic properties of the drugs. In other words, taking twice as much aspirin as the label on the bottle instructs does not make the patient feel twice as well, nor does it speed relief to the aching body part in half the time.

Common Side Effects

Nonprescription painkillers can produce severe side effects. Because aspirin and other NSAID drugs block COX-1, they inhibit the production of the mucus that provides a protective lining to the stomach and intestines. Therefore, overuse of the NSAID drugs can cause upset stomachs and even bleeding in the stomach and intestines.

The dangers of overuse of acetaminophen are well chronicled: Overdosing on the drug could damage the liver. The function of the liver is to store vitamins, sugars, and fats from foods and use them to manufacture proteins and other vital chemicals in the body. The liver also breaks down and neutralizes substances that are harmful to the body, such as alcohol.

When blood containing acetaminophen passes through the liver, the organ secretes a toxic by-product from the drug that tends to stay in the liver and kill healthy liver cells. If the liver is bombarded by too many doses of acetaminophen, the organ can become overwhelmed by the toxic by-products and fall victim to acute liver failure, which can occur within a few days. Acute liver failure is often a fatal condition. A joint study by the Universities of Texas and Washington found that acetaminophen overdoses are responsible for more than half the acute liver failure cases in the United States.

Rebound Headaches

Side effects are not the only possible problems associated with the use of painkillers. Headache sufferers who take too many painkillers may find the pills stop working and that to get the desired effect they have to take more and more painkillers. As a result, the painkillers wear off quickly and the headaches return. These are known as rebound headaches. Doctors are not sure why nonprescription painkillers stop working from overuse, but they suspect that the body's natural pain-fighting abilities break down when they are bombarded by too many painkillers.

Teenagers, whose abuse of nonprescription painkillers is believed to be widespread, often suffer from rebound headaches. In one study by the Cleveland Clinic, 22 percent of adolescents who were treated in the institution's pediatric headache center were found to be overdosing on nonprescription painkillers—meaning they took at least 4 doses a week for more than 6 weeks. One patient whose habits were measured by the study averaged 28 doses a week. "Three times a week is probably excessive," says David Dodick, a neurologist at a Mayo Clinic facility in Arizona. "They need better headache management."[18]

> A joint study by the Universities of Texas and Washington found that acetaminophen overdoses are responsible for more than half the acute liver failure cases in the United States.

Moreover, overdosing on over-the-counter painkillers for injuries to ankles or other parts of the body could also cause rebound headaches. Jesus Eric Peña-Garza, a headache specialist at Vanderbilt University Medical Center in Tennessee, says he has treated patients for severe headaches who acknowledged overdosing on nonprescription painkillers to treat sprained ankles and other sports-related injuries. Although they may think they are speeding pain relief to their sore ankles, he says, they are also laying the foundation for rebound headaches. Adds Stanford University neurology professor Paul Graham Fisher, "I can't tell you how many times I have a family in my office, and the parents say, 'Oh, that's where all the ibuprofens are going.' Kids think it's OK to take eight, ten or fifteen a day. It's over-the-counter so what could be wrong with it?"[19]

A Lifetime of Pain

As their bodies adjust to painkillers, many people find that over-the-counter remedies stop giving them any relief at all. Many of these people face a lifetime of pain, since doctors are not likely to prescribe opiate-based painkillers because these headaches are not caused by traumatic head injures, cancer, or other debilitating illnesses. Therefore, they have no alterative than to endure their headaches until they go away on their own.

That's what happened to Elizabeth Pirsch, a 48-year-old attorney from Alexandria, Virginia, who started suffering headaches at the age of 6. She took over-the-counter medication intended to relieve nasal congestion caused by colds and flu. The product contains acetaminophen. "I remember lying in bed and crying and wishing someone would cut off my head because it hurt so much,"[20] says Pirsch.

By the time she reached her thirties, Pirsch was unable to find relief in over-the-counter medications. Meanwhile, her headaches had grown worse and were now regarded to be of migraine caliber. In addition to severe headaches, Pirsch also suffered from chronic pains in her shoulders caused, she believes, by overmedicating herself. Says Richard Lipton, a neurologist at Albert Einstein College of Medicine in New York, "The pain mechanisms in the body adapt to having pain medicines on board."[21]

New Research, New Concerns

Scientists continue to turn up evidence suggesting that some painkillers could have detrimental effects on humans. In 2008 tests indicated that a drug known as rimonabant causes memory loss in laboratory animals. Rimonabant is prescribed as a diet drug, but since the medication provides an anti-inflammatory effect it has been prescribed for pain as well. Rimonabant has not been licensed for use in America but is widely prescribed in Europe. Given the test findings, it is unlikely the Food and Drug Administration will permit the use of the drug in America.

As new evidence surfaces about the dangers of common painkillers such as aspirin and acetaminophen, doctors urge patients to use common sense when taking the pills—perhaps, they suggest, a mild headache should be treated with rest rather than a double dose of a nonprescription analgesic. As for the abusers of opiate-based painkillers, many face uncertain lives of addiction. Sam Rayburn says he is lucky to have been caught—his arrest led to his rehabilitation. Otherwise, he says, "I think it would have led me to either jail or to death—I don't think there was really any other option."[22]

What Are the Dangers of Painkillers?

Primary Source Quotes

66 **Pharmaceuticals such as OxyContin can be diverted in many ways. The most popular form is known as 'doctor shopping,' where individuals, who may or may not have legitimate illnesses requiring a doctor's prescription for controlled substances, visit many doctors to acquire large amounts of controlled substances.** 99

—U.S. Drug Enforcement Administration, "OxyContin: Description/Overview," August 2006. www.usdoj.gov.

The U.S. Drug Enforcement Administration enforces federal laws that regulate illegal drug use and trafficking.

66 **Detecting drug abusers is not always easy, and while physicians and nurses want to relieve suffering, we have to be careful that our efforts to treat legitimate pain do not end up feeding addictions.** 99

—Victoria McEvoy, "A Doctor's Dilemma: Prescribing Pain Pills Is Getting Trickier," *Boston Globe*, February 4, 2008. www.boston.com.

McEvoy is the medical director of Massachusetts General West Medical Group and a professor of pediatrics at Harvard University Medical School.

* Editor's Note: While the definition of a primary source can be narrowly or broadly defined, for the purposes of Compact Research, a primary source consists of: 1) results of original research presented by an organization or researcher; 2) eyewitness accounts of events, personal experience, or work experience; 3) first-person editorials offering pundits' opinions; 4) government officials presenting political plans and/or policies; 5) representatives of organizations presenting testimony or policy.

66Acetaminophen is one of the most commonly used drugs in the United States yet it is also an important cause of serious liver injury. . . . Taking more than the recommended amount can cause liver damage, ranging from abnormalities in liver function blood tests, to acute liver failure, and even death. Many cases of overdose are caused by patients inadvertently taking more than the recommended dose.**99**

—U.S. Food and Drug Administration, "Joint Meeting of the Drug Safety and Risk Management Advisory Committee with the Anesthetic and Life Support Drugs Advisory Committee and the Nonprescription Drugs Advisory Committee," June 29–30, 2009. www.fda.gov.

The U.S. Food and Drug Administration enacts regulations governing the use and sale of prescription and nonprescription drugs in America.

66There is universal agreement on the safety of acetaminophen when used as directed on the label. We know that the overwhelming majority of adults use this product safely and that the majority of serious adverse events related to unintentional acetaminophen overdose are associated with prescription medicines containing acetaminophen.**99**

—Linda A. Suydam, "Statement from the Consumer Healthcare Products Association on Today's Joint FDA Advisory Committee Recommendations on Over-the-Counter Medicines Containing Acetaminophen," *Consumer Healthcare Products Association*, June 30, 2009. www.chpa-info.org.

Suydam is president of the Consumer Healthcare Products Association, a trade association that represents manufacturers of nonprescription painkillers.

66Most painkillers on the pharmaceutical market today are central nervous system depressants. That means they decrease the ability of the brain and circuit of nerves throughout the body to do their job. No matter how much I willed my body to do what I wanted, it had already lost the ability to respond.**99**

—Tony Mandarich, *My Dirty Little Secrets—Steroids, Alcohol and God: The Tony Mandarich Story.* Ann Arbor, MI: Modern History, 2009.

Mandarich is a former NFL lineman whose career was cut short by prescription painkiller abuse.

❝Pain is part of the game. It's as much a part of the game as the crowds or the Miller Lite commercials or the TV cameras. If you can't endure the pain, you can't play in the NFL.❞

—Jerome Bettis, *The Bus: My Life In and Out of a Helmet.* New York: Doubleday, 2007.

Bettis is a former NFL running back.

❝I'll admit that pain is a difficult thing to measure, and I am sure that the majority of my patients have real pain. But some of them are just plain junkies, and junkies will say or do just about anything to get high.❞

—Dustin Ballard, "Jackson Not Alone in Overuse of Painkillers," *Marin Independent Journal,* July 5, 2009. www.marinij.com.

Ballard is an emergency room physician in San Rafael, California.

❝Pain medications suppress the brain's own pain-fighting substances . . . and sensitize the nerve cells of the brain so that head pain recurs when the patient stops taking the pain medicine. And if the sufferer does not continue taking the medications on a regular basis, the headache comes back: a true 'vicious cycle.'❞

—Robert S. Kunkel, *Headaches: A Cleveland Clinic Handbook.* Cleveland, OH: Cleveland Clinic, 2007.

Kunkel is a consulting physician at the Cleveland Clinic Neurological Center for Pain in Ohio.

❝Teens are abusing prescription drugs because many believe the myth that these drugs provide a 'safe' high and they are easily available.❞

—White House Office of National Drug Control Policy, *Prescription for Danger: A Report on the Troubling Trend of Prescription and Over-the-Counter Drug Abuse Among the Nation's Teens,* January 2008. www.theantidrug.com.

The White House Office of National Drug Control Policy coordinates the activities of several federal drug agencies and helps formulate policies to control drug addiction and trafficking in America.

Facts and Illustrations

What Are the Dangers of Painkillers?

- A drug dealer arrested in Burlington, Vermont, told police that he sold between **90 and 150 OxyContin pills a day**, earning a profit of some **$1.5 million** over a period of 6 months.

- About **2 percent** of young people between the ages of 12 and 17, or about 5.2 million teenagers, are believed to abuse prescription painkillers, according to the Substance Abuse and Mental Health Services Administration.

- **Eighteen percent** of teenage painkiller abusers consume them at least weekly.

- Every day about **2,500 young people** abuse prescription painkillers for the first time.

- Sixty percent of teens who abuse prescription painkillers take their first doses **before the age of 15**.

- The prescription painkillers that are most commonly abused by young people are **OxyContin**, which contains the opioid oxycodone, and **Vicodin**, which contains acetaminophen and the opioid hydrocodone.

- About **325,000 people a year** are hospitalized after they overdose on prescription painkillers.

More Young People Inititate Drug Use with Painkillers

Marijuana used to be the first drug tried by most young people experimenting with drugs, but now prescription painkillers hold that distinction. According to 2007 statistics compiled by the Substance Abuse and Mental Health Services Administration, more than 2.1 million people over the age of 12 try painkillers as their "initiate" drug, meaning the first drug they try. Marijuana still holds second place, with just over 2 million initiates a year.

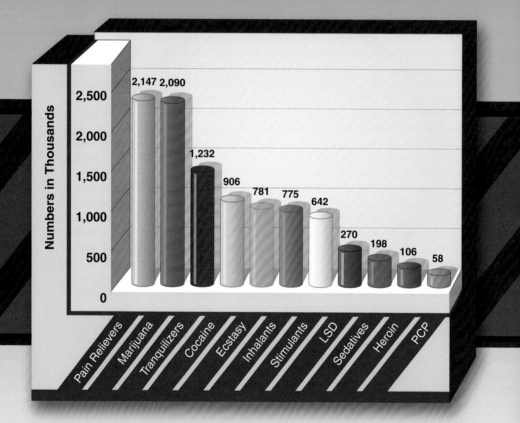

Source: Substance Abuse and Mental Health Services Administration, *Results from the 2007 National Survey on Drug Use and Health: National Findings*, September 2008. www.oas.samhsa.gov.

- A **third to half** of all adults are believed to consume doses of non-prescription painkillers in excess of the maximum amounts recommended on the labels; about **1.5 percent** of those abusers suffer from rebound headaches.

How Young People Obtain Painkillers

Stealing painkillers from the medicine cabinet at home is known as "pharming." More than 50 percent of young people who abuse painkillers obtain them from friends or relatives, according to 2007 statistics compiled by the White House Office of National Drug Control Policy. Nearly 20 percent of young abusers say they can obtain the pills from doctors, although drug experts believe most of those painkillers are obtained illegally by teens using other people's prescriptions. About 5 percent of young painkiller abusers say they take the pills from friends or relatives—typically parents—without asking.

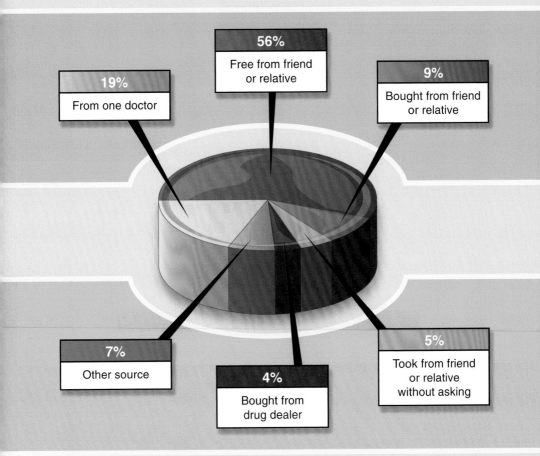

56%
Free from friend or relative

19%
From one doctor

9%
Bought from friend or relative

7%
Other source

4%
Bought from drug dealer

5%
Took from friend or relative without asking

Source: White House Office of National Drug Control Policy, *Prescription for Danger: A Report on the Troubling Trend of Prescription and Over-the-Counter Drug Abuse Among the Nation's Teens*, January 2008. www.theantidrug.com.

Study on Abuse of Nonprescription Painkillers

Researchers in Colorado and Australia conducted a joint study of 127 dental clinic patients to find out whether they were exceeding the recommended maximum dosages of their nonprescription painkillers. The study found that 22 of the 127 patients regularly exceeded the dosages recommended by the labels. Fourteen of the patients reported taking as much as 12,000 milligrams of ibuprofen a day—10 times the recommended maximum dosage. Five of the naproxen users often tripled the maximum recommended dosages while 3 of the acetaminophen users said they often doubled the recommended dosages. People who overdose on ibuprofen and naproxen risk damaging their stomachs and intestines while overuse of acetaminophen could cause acute liver failure, which could be fatal.

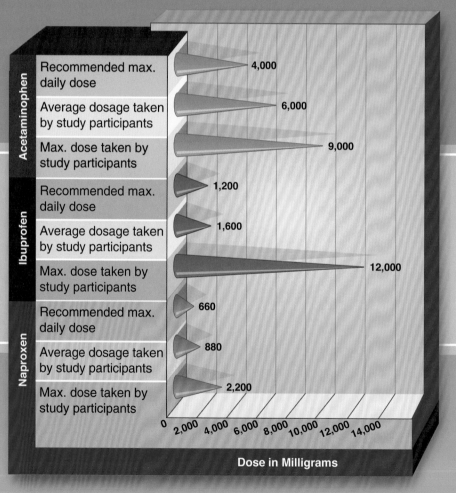

		Dose in Milligrams
Acetaminophen	Recommended max. daily dose	4,000
	Average dosage taken by study participants	6,000
	Max. dose taken by study participants	9,000
Ibuprofen	Recommended max. daily dose	1,200
	Average dosage taken by study participants	1,600
	Max. dose taken by study participants	12,000
Naproxen	Recommended max. daily dose	660
	Average dosage taken by study participants	880
	Max. dose taken by study participants	2,200

Source: Kennon J. Heard et al., "Overuse of Nonprescription Analgesics by Dental Clinic Participants," BMC Oral Health, December 9, 2008. www.biomedical.com.

Hydrocodone Is the Most Abused Prescription Painkiller

young people and others turn to prescription painkillers to get high,
most frequently abuse Vicodin, Lortab, and Lorcet, which contain
codone. According to the Substance Abuse and Mental Health
ces Administration, nearly half of first-time prescription painkiller
ers use Vicodin as the "initiate drug." Other popular initiate drugs are
ol 3, Darvocet, and Darvon, which contain codeine, and Percocet,
contains oxycodone.

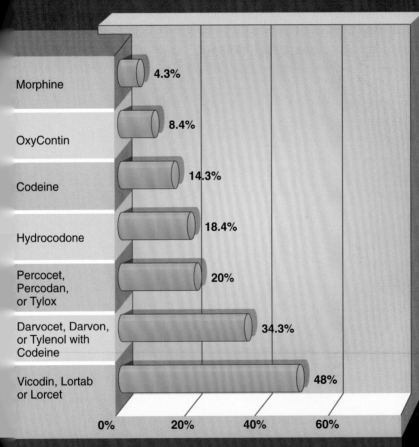

Drug	Percentage
Morphine	4.3%
OxyContin	8.4%
Codeine	14.3%
Hydrocodone	18.4%
Percocet, Percodan, or Tylox	20%
Darvocet, Darvon, or Tylenol with Codeine	34.3%
Vicodin, Lortab or Lorcet	48%

0%   20%   40%   60%

Percentage of First-Time Abusers Using Drug

ubstance Abuse and Mental Health Services Administration, "Nonmedical Users of Pain Relievers: Characteristics
t Initiatives," *National Survey on Drug Use and Health Report,* 2006. www.oas.samhsa.gov.

How Effective Is Government Oversight of Painkillers?

66Vioxx is a terrible tragedy and a profound regulatory failure. I would argue that the FDA, as currently configured, is incapable of protecting America against another Vioxx.99

—David Graham, FDA scientist who first raised concerns about the safety of the prescription painkiller Vioxx.

66Make no mistake. [The] FDA is only as good as its workforce, and its current workforce is unsurpassed. Our scientists and medical officers and consumer safety officers are second to none.99

—Andrew C. von Eschenbach, former commissioner of the FDA.

The Power of the FDA

The U.S. Food and Drug Administration (FDA) is the federal agency charged with regulating the sales of prescription and nonprescription drugs in America. The actual testing of the drugs is conducted by the manufacturers before they go on the market, but the results of those tests are turned over to the FDA, which assesses the results and decides whether to approve the sales of the drugs to American consumers. Even after painkillers and other drugs have been approved for the market, though, concerns about safety often arise—perhaps even years or decades after their initial approvals. In such cases the FDA can order that warnings to consumers be included on the labels for the drugs. In some cases the agency has ordered drugs withdrawn from the market.

As evidence mounted that abuse of nonprescription painkillers could cause severe health consequences such as stomach bleeding, liver failure, and even death, the FDA acted to make consumers aware of the dangers. In 2009 the agency directed manufacturers of acetaminophen and the NSAIDs—ibuprofen, aspirin, and naproxen—to include very specific warning labels on their products, informing consumers of the dangers of overdosing. Charles Ganley, director of nonprescription drugs in the FDA's Center for Drug Evaluation and Research, said:

> Acetaminophen and the NSAIDs are commonly used drugs for both children and adults because they are effective in reducing fevers and relieving minor aches and pain, such as headaches and muscle aches. . . . However, the risks associated with their use need to be clearly identified on the label so that consumers taking these drugs are fully aware of the potential harm they can cause. It is important that they know how to take these medications safely to reduce their risk.[23]

The new labels include language specifically warning consumers of acetaminophen that overuse of the drug could cause liver damage, and the labels for the NSAIDs include warnings about stomach bleeding. The new labeling requirements mandated by the FDA illustrate the regulatory power the federal agency holds over the American drug industry.

Clinical Trials

Before a painkiller is approved for human consumption, it has to go through a research and development process that often takes several years. It is likely that the drug will undergo all manner of tests in the labs, including trials on lab animals. When the drug company feels the new substance is ready for testing on humans, it will apply to the FDA to perform what are known as clinical trials. In most cases new drugs must undergo three phases of clinical trials before they will be approved for public consumption.

In phase 1 a small group of volunteers—usually no more than 80—

will be given the drug. This small group is likely to include some patients, but many healthy volunteers will receive the drug as well. Doctors will study their reactions to the drug, particularly any side effects the drug may prompt.

> " The new labels include language specifically warning consumers of acetaminophen that overuse of the drug could cause liver damage, and the labels for the NSAIDs include warnings about stomach bleeding. "

In phase 2 the substance will be given to patients whose conditions are specifically addressed by the experimental drug. Phase 2 trials may include several hundred participants. Many of the participants will, without their knowledge, receive placebos, which are fake drugs that have no effect on the patient's condition. People who receive placebos do not know they are receiving fake drugs. They serve in what is known as the control group so that the reactions of those who receive the drugs can be measured against those who do not.

Phase 3 trials include a few thousand participants. Again, the drug company is studying the reactions to the drug by the participants. It could take several years before a drug completes testing in all three clinical trial phases.

At the conclusion of phase 3, the results are submitted to the FDA, which performs a cost-benefit analysis of the drug—the agency recognizes the drug may be harmful to some people under certain circumstances, but its wider benefit to patients who are ailing and in pain are weighed against those costs. Finally, the FDA makes the ultimate decision about whether to approve the release of the drug to American consumers.

The Vioxx Debacle

When the COX inhibitor Vioxx was approved by the FDA in 1999, it was regarded as much stronger than other well-known COX inhibitors such as aspirin, ibuprofen, and acetaminophen. And since Vioxx blocked only COX-2, it was considered much gentler on the stomach than the nonprescription drugs.

Vioxx, available only by prescription, was found to be particularly effective for arthritis patients, whose pain is chronic and often debilitating. Eventually, doctors would write some 92 million prescriptions for Vioxx.

Within a year, though, evidence surfaced showing that Vioxx doubled the chances of heart attack and stroke in some patients. The FDA responded by requiring Vioxx's manufacturer, Merck, to include new warning labels on the bottles, alerting patients to the dangers. Meanwhile, evidence continued to mount that Vioxx was harmful, and in 2004 Merck was forced to withdraw Vioxx from the market.

Studies have shown that inhibiting COX-2 tends to force blood cell components known as platelets to stick together. These sticky platelets form clumps that can block arteries, causing heart attacks and strokes. Inhibiting COX-2 in healthy people does not have much of an effect on their arteries, but for people already at risk for heart attack or stroke, the extra clumping action promoted by Vioxx could be fatal. By the time Merck withdrew the drug from the market, it was estimated that more than 27,000 people who were taking Vioxx died of heart attacks or strokes.

Criticism of the FDA

Since the truth about Vioxx surfaced, the FDA has fallen under intense criticism by members of Congress for failing to recognize the dangers of Vioxx—particularly after evidence surfaced that some FDA scientists suspected the new drug was dangerous but their opinions were ignored by the agency's administrators. One FDA scientist, David Graham, said that after he raised concerns about Vioxx, he was told by his supervisors to keep quiet. "I was warned that if I persisted in this fashion, there would be serious consequences for me,"[24] Graham said.

The scientist eventually took his concerns to Congress and is credited with being in-

> **Before a painkiller is approved for human consumption, it has to go through a research and development process that often takes several years.**

strumental in the campaign to force the withdrawal of Vioxx from the marketplace. Said Representative Edward J. Markey of Massachusetts, "The spotlight is now shining on the FDA more than any other federal agency as one in need of reform."[25]

Fees for Tests

Critics of the FDA believe the agency's failure to detect the dangers of Vioxx can be traced to the Prescription Drug User Fee Act, a law passed in 1992 that provides fees to the FDA to assess the effectiveness and dangers of new drugs. The fees, which can total in the hundreds of millions of dollars, are paid by the drug companies that submit applications for new drugs to the FDA.

> Since the truth about Vioxx surfaced, the FDA has fallen under intense criticism by members of Congress for failing to recognize the dangers of Vioxx—particularly after evidence surfaced that some FDA scientists suspected the new drug was dangerous but their opinions were ignored by the agency's administrators.

According to Marcia Angell, a senior lecturer at Harvard University Medical School in Massachusetts and a harsh critic of the FDA, the drug companies should not be paying the FDA to assess the safety of the drugs—a situation she says makes it difficult for the federal agency to serve as an independent monitor. "That puts the FDA on the payroll of the industry it regulates, and makes it more likely that drugs will be reviewed favorably—a bargain for the drug companies,"[26] she insists.

In 2007, in light of the Vioxx debacle, Congress looked closely at the operation of the FDA. Instead of giving the agency an independent source of funding, though, lawmakers hiked the fees on the drug companies by about 25 percent. The increased fees are intended to give the FDA more personnel to assess the effectiveness and safety of drugs. One facet of the new law governing the FDA gives the agency the power to order new clinical trials even after drugs are already on the market. Such tests could provide an ongoing assessment of the drugs that could better reveal long-term effects that do not show up in phases 1, 2, or 3.

Also, under the changes approved by Congress, the drug companies must publicly disclose the results of

> " In 2007, in light of the Vioxx debacle, Congress looked closely at the operation of the FDA. "

clinical trials and other tests. After Vioxx had been approved, reports surfaced suggesting that Merck tailored its clinical trials to emphasize the benefits and minimize the risks and that the FDA should have done a better job of detecting the bias in the tests.

Black Box Warnings

The Vioxx fiasco has also made the FDA much more cautious about painkillers. After Merck withdrew Vioxx from the market, the FDA looked closely at a similar COX-2 inhibitor, Bextra, which was distributed by a Merck competitor, Pfizer. In 2005, at the request of the FDA, Pfizer withdrew Bextra from the market. A third COX-2 inhibitor, Celebrex—which is also distributed by Pfizer—has also raised questions among patients who have suffered heart attacks and strokes while using the drug.

Despite the possible dangers of taking Celebrex, the drug remains available to arthritis patients and others in chronic pain. To keep the drug on the market, Pfizer agreed to include a so-called black box warning on the side of the bottle. The black box warning is the strictest warning that a drug can carry; as the name suggests, the warning is surrounded by a bold, black border designed to catch the eye of the consumer. Inside the black box the warning urges patients to take the drug in the lowest dose possible.

Off-Label Uses

The FDA's new vigilance has also extended to opioid painkillers. In 2009 the agency contacted two dozen American drug companies that manufacture opiate-based painkillers to develop an industry-wide plan to cut down on overdoses of Percocet, Vicodin, and similar drugs. The final plan is expected to include new warning labels for the bottles and new guidelines for doctors, refining their instructions on how much of the medication is needed to reduce pain. The new policy is also expected to address doctors who prescribe painkillers for so-called off-label uses—in other words, to treat conditions for which the painkiller is not specifically intended.

Off-label use of pain medication is seen as a major reason some people overdose—people do not know the proper doses to take, and their doctors may just be guessing at the proper amounts to prescribe. The tendency by doctors to prescribe painkillers for off-label uses may have been in reaction to the trend that started in the 1990s when pharmaceutical companies as well as advocates for pain management stepped up pressure on doctors to alleviate pain as part of their patients' treatments.

> **Off-label use of pain medication is seen as a major reason some people overdose—people do not know the proper doses to take, and their doctors may just be guessing at the proper amounts to prescribe.**

In 2007 three people died after taking the painkiller Fentora, which is composed of fentanyl, an opiate believed to be 80 times stronger than morphine. After their deaths it was determined that doctors prescribed Fentora to the patients for off-label uses. (A fourth patient committed suicide by taking an overdose of Fentora, apparently obtaining the drug from somebody other than a doctor). Fentora is a particularly strong opioid; it is intended for cancer patients who are already taking other opiate-based painkillers yet still feeling significant pain. This is not an unusual side effect for many cancer patients—they build up resistance to their opiate-based painkillers and must turn to stronger drugs to find relief. More potent than morphine, Fentora is approved by the FDA for patients who cannot find relief with milder opiates, and, in fact, the agency has specified that it is to be prescribed to cancer patients only.

In the cases of the four deaths, though, investigators found that none of the patients had cancer—in fact, two were suffering from migraine headaches and had no previous history of taking opiate-based painkillers. Since the patients had not built up resistance to opiate-based drugs, their bodies could not handle the jolt delivered by Fentora, and they died of respiratory failure.

FDA Missteps

The federal government has monitored the sales and uses of painkillers since 1906, when Congress passed the U.S. Pure Food and Drug Act. Since then Congress has constantly refined and enacted new laws designed to protect Americans from dangerous drugs.

Still, the system is far from perfect. The FDA's missteps on Vioxx have prompted critics to call for the reform of the FDA. Proposals include providing the agency with an independent source of funding so that it will not be using money paid by the drug industry to assess products the drug industry intends to sell to pain sufferers and other patients. Angell maintains this step is important in order for the FDA to closely monitor the drug industry to ensure that only safe drugs are approved for consumption by Americans. Says Angell, "The scrutiny that this agency exists to provide is vital to our health."[27]

How Effective Is Government Oversight of Painkillers?

> **It is time to restore the FDA to its purpose, which is to protect the public from unsafe food, drugs, and devices, not to accommodate the industries it regulates.**

—Marcia Angell, "Charting a New Course for the FDA," *Boston Globe*, April 6, 2009. www.boston.com.

Angell is a senior lecturer at Harvard University Medical School in Massachusetts and the author of the book *The Truth About the Drug Companies: How They Deceive Us and What to Do About It.*

> **The FDA holds itself to the highest possible standard—perfection. While we know that perfect is not possible for mere mortals, it is the goal we must strive for. The men and women of the FDA know that safeguarding the health and well-being of the American public is a zero-defects operation. There is no margin for error—because when errors occur, people may die.**

—Andrew C. von Eschenbach, "The FDA's Blueprint for Change," June 10, 2008. www.fda.gov.

Von Eschenbach is the former commissioner of the FDA.

Bracketed quotes indicate conflicting positions.

* Editor's Note: While the definition of a primary source can be narrowly or broadly defined, for the purposes of Compact Research, a primary source consists of: 1) results of original research presented by an organization or researcher; 2) eyewitness accounts of events, personal experience, or work experience; 3) first-person editorials offering pundits' opinions; 4) government officials presenting political plans and/or policies; 5) representatives of organizations presenting testimony or policy.

"Drug development faces major challenges. Research and development expenditures are increasing at a rate far exceeding that for new product approvals. Safety concerns have made regulators more cautious about the drugs they approve. Public anxiety has increased."

—Tufts Center for the Study of Drug Development, *Outlook 2006*, 2006. http:// csdd.tufts.edu.

The Tufts Center for the Study of Drug Development, based at Tufts University in Massachusetts, examines issues related to the development and safety of new drugs.

"The regulatory threshold for the approval of new drugs should be higher if there are safe and [effective] alternatives already in existence. Given the magnitude of the problem and the danger to public health, it is imperative that these measures be implemented as soon as possible, and that the public be made aware of the dangers associated with using new drugs."

—Shoo K. Lee, "Re-Examining Our Approach to the Approval and Use of New Drugs," *Canadian Medical Association Journal*, June 20, 2006.

Lee is a professor of pediatrics at the University of Alberta in Canada.

"Lawsuits are presently swirling around both the physicians who prescribed [Vioxx] and the manufacturer. I have always felt that if a drug was FDA-approved and I understood and explained the side effects to my patients, I could feel confident that my decision to write the prescription was safe. Now, I am not so sure."

—Zoe Diana Draelos, "How Safe Is Safe? *Dermatology Times*, October 2007.

Draelos is an associate professor of dermatology at Wake Forest University School of Medicine in North Carolina.

> 66 Merck couldn't advertise Vioxx—a painkiller origi-
> nally approved to treat rheumatoid arthritis—to treat
> tennis elbow, but doctors were free to prescribe it to
> anybody they pleased. By the time Vioxx was pulled
> from the market, it was estimated to have killed more
> Americans than were killed in the Korean War. 99

—Shannon Brownlee, "Newtered," *Washington Monthly*, October 2007.

Brownlee is a senior fellow at the New America Foundation, a Washington, D.C.–
based institution that examines health care and other public policy issues, and
the author of *Overtreated: Why Too Much Medicine Is Making Us Sicker and
Poorer.*

> 66 Vioxx, Ketek, Avandia, Paxil—these drugs have harmed
> families across our country and come to symbolize the
> urgent need for reform. Families should never have
> to play 'Rx Roulette' when they reach into their medi-
> cine cabinets. 99

—Edward J. Markey, "Committee Takes Important Action on Drug Approval Process," June 21, 2007.
http://markey.house.gov.

Markey represents Massachusetts in Congress and is a sponsor of legislation to
reform the FDA.

> 66 Finally, the Food and Drug Administration is propos-
> ing to put labels on over-the-counter pain relievers
> warning of the potential for stomach bleeding and
> liver damage. Our major question is: What took the
> agency so long? 99

—Peter Lurie, "FDA Proposal for Painkillers Is Decades Late," Public Citizen, December 19, 2006. www.citizen.org.

Lurie is deputy director of health research for Public Citizen, a Washington,
D.C.–based consumer advocacy group.

How Effective Is Government Oversight of Painkillers?

- Despite concerns that Celebrex causes heart attacks and stroke, the Cox-2 inhibitor's sales total more than **$2 billion** a year.

- In 2008 Pfizer paid **$894 million** to more than 8,000 people who claimed to have suffered heart attacks or strokes after taking Celebrex.

- In one clinical study of Vioxx, **21 out of 1,000** volunteers developed stomach ailments, and **45 out of 1,000** volunteers taking naproxen suffered from stomach problems.

- Doctors wrote more than **92 million** prescriptions for Vioxx before it was withdrawn from the market in 2004.

- To settle claims that Vioxx had caused heart attacks and stroke, drug manufacturer Merck agreed to pay nearly **$5 billion** to some 44,000 Vioxx users or their survivors; the average payment was about $200,000, although some people received as much as $1.5 million.

- After Congress hiked the fees drug companies must pay to the FDA in 2007, the agency added some **1,300 biologists and chemists** to its staff to help assess the safety of drugs sold in America.

- According to the *Wall Street Journal*, **80 percent** of patients who take the opioid painkiller Actiq (a potent narcotic intended for use by cancer patients) received their prescriptions off-label, meaning for conditions for which the painkiller is not specifically intended.

Amount of Tylenol Consumed by Americans

The U.S. Food and Drug Administration believes people take too much acetaminophen, a habit that could result in liver damage. In 2009, the agency considered a recommendation by an advisory board to slash the maximum recommended dosage of acetaminophen from 4,000 milligrams to 2,600 milligrams. On the American market, the most familiar brand that contains acetaminophen is Tylenol. Statistics show that Americans spend hundreds of millions of dollars a year on the 3 most popular versions of the product, which include Tylenol, Tylenol PM, and Tylenol Arthritis.

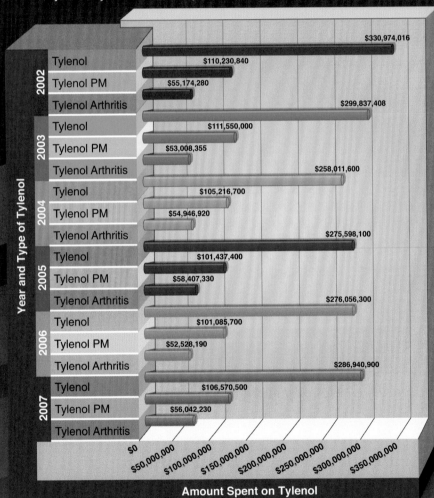

Year and Type of Tylenol

2002
- Tylenol: $330,974,016
- Tylenol PM: $110,230,840
- Tylenol Arthritis: $55,174,280

2003
- Tylenol: $299,837,408
- Tylenol PM: $111,550,000
- Tylenol Arthritis: $53,008,355

2004
- Tylenol: $258,011,600
- Tylenol PM: $105,216,700
- Tylenol Arthritis: $54,946,920

2005
- Tylenol: $275,598,100
- Tylenol PM: $101,437,400
- Tylenol Arthritis: $58,407,330

2006
- Tylenol: $276,056,300
- Tylenol PM: $101,085,700
- Tylenol Arthritis: $52,528,190

2007
- Tylenol: $286,940,900
- Tylenol PM: $106,570,500
- Tylenol Arthritis: $56,042,230

$0, $50,000,000, $100,000,000, $150,000,000, $200,000,000, $250,000,000, $300,000,000, $350,000,000

Amount Spent on Tylenol

Sources: Marina Marketos, "Top 200 OTC/HBC Brands in 2002," *Drug Topics*, February 17, 2003. http://licence.icopyright.net; Sandra Levy, "Top 200 OTC/HBC Brands in 2003," *Drug Topics*, June 7, 2004. http://drugtopics.modernmedicine.com; *Drug Topics*, "Top 200 OTC/HBC Brands in 2004," *Drug Topics*, April 18, 2005. http://drugtopics.modernmedicine.com; "Top 200 OTC/HBC Brands in 2005," *Drug Topics*, April 17, 2006. http://drugtopics.modernmedicine.com; "Top 200 OTC/HBC Brands in 2006," *Drug Topics*, May 7, 2007. http://drugtopics.modernmedicine.com; "Top 200 OTC/HBC Brands in 2007," *Drug Topics*, February 25, 2008. http://drugtopics.modernmedicine.com.

Bringing a New Drug to Market Costs $1.2 Billion

It often costs about $1.2 billion to bring a new drug to market. Typically, new drugs spend eight years in clinical trials that could cost their developers $600 million or more. Meanwhile, drug companies spend hundreds of millions of dollars in the laboratory, or preclinical, phase while spending hundreds of millions more in company time and resources to develop the drug.

Cost to develop a new biopharmaceutical surpasses $1 billion

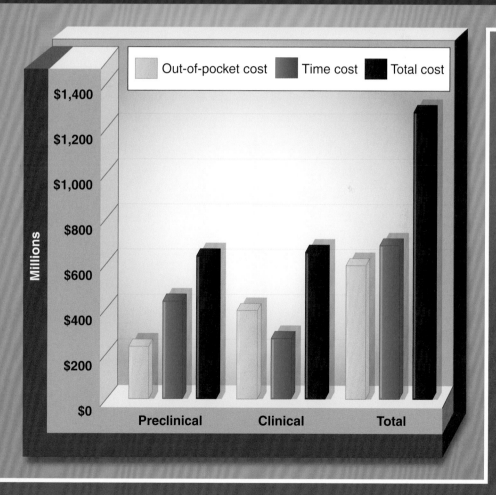

Source: Tufts Center for the Study of Drug Development, *Outlook 2008*, 2008. www.csdd.tufts.edu.

The FDA's Budget for Assessing Drugs Expands

In 2003 and 2004, before Vioxx was pulled off the market, the FDA spent about $400 million a year assessing the safety of new drugs proposed for human consumption in the United States. In 2007, in response to the FDA's failures to detect the hazards of taking Vioxx, Congress assessed higher fees on drug makers to help the FDA expand its investigatory role. In 2009, the FDA budgeted more than $700 million to investigate the safety of new drugs—much of the increase funded by the higher fees on drug makers. To help detect defects in new drugs, the FDA expanded its staff of chemists and biologists by 1,300 employees.

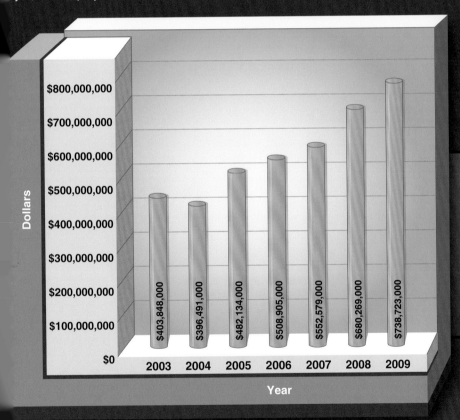

Sources: U.S. Food and Drug Administration, "FY 2007 Budget Summary," May 27, 2009; "FY 2008 Budget Summary"; FY 2009 Congressional Justification. www.fda.gov.

- According to the American Pain Foundation, in 2008 the FDA approved just **one pain medication** for human consumption—Durezol, a medication administered to reduce pain following eye surgery.

- In 2009 an FDA advisory panel recommended the agency ban the opiate-based painkillers Vicodin and Percocet due to their adverse effects on the human liver; each year some **9 million** prescriptions are written for Percocet, and doctors write more than **100 million** prescriptions a year for Vicodin.

- By 2009, versions of **38 prescription painkillers** carried FDA-mandated **black box warnings**.

- According to CenterWatch, a Boston publishing company that monitors the progress of drug development, during 2009 at least **480 experimental pain drugs** were in clinical trials in America.

Are There Alternatives to Using Painkillers?

> **I'm very sick—I suffer from an inoperable brain tumor, a seizure disorder, life-threatening wasting syndrome, severe chronic pain and other documented medical conditions, but I'll be damned if I'm going to let the federal government prohibit me from improving my health with cannabis.**
>
> —Angel Raich, a California woman who sued the U.S. Justice Department to legalize the use of marijuana for medicinal purposes.

> **Marijuana has a high potential for abuse, has no currently accepted use in treatment in the United States, and has a lack of accepted safety for use under medical supervision.**
>
> —David Satcher, former U.S. surgeon general.

Living Pain Free Without Painkillers

People who suffer from pain can often find relief without the need to take painkillers. Patients with minor aches may find that exercising or making other changes in their lifestyles can help make them healthier and therefore less likely to be in pain. There are also ways in which chronic-pain patients can find relief without drugs. Chiropractors, physical therapists, and massage therapists can often help make pain go away by manipulating bones and muscles.

There are many alternative therapies available to people in pain, including acupuncture, aromatherapy, and hypnosis. Doctors are dubious about the effectiveness of alternative therapies, but they often do not discourage patients from trying them. Most doctors believe patients are better off if they can find ways to manage pain that do not require them to swallow massive doses of painkilling drugs.

One alternative therapy is hypnosis, in which a trained professional—often a psychologist—will lead the patient into a deep state of relaxation, then plant a hypnotic suggestion into his or her mind. The technique is often employed to help people give up smoking—the hypnotist will plant a notion with the smoker suggesting that smoking is repugnant. In the case of a patient who suffers from pain, the hypnotic suggestion may raise the patient's threshold for pain.

> " **Doctors are dubious about the effectiveness of alternative therapies, but they often do not discourage patients from trying them.** "

Henry Polic II, a movie and TV actor, suffers from skin cancer. He undergoes radiation treatments, which cause burning pain on his skin. After several painful radiation treatments, Polic visited a hypnotherapist, whose treatments have helped him use the power of his mind to overcome the pain. While under hypnosis Polic imagines himself reliving a pleasant vacation in Florida. According to Polic, the pain he suffers from the radiation treatments is a lot more bearable while he is under hypnosis. "I was never a skeptic of hypnosis, but I'm amazed at what a difference it has made,"[28] he says.

Physical Therapy Can Reduce Pain

Many doctors regard drugs as only one part of the patient's therapy and will refer the patient to a physical therapist or other pain specialist. A physical therapist is a professional who helps people recover from physical disabilities caused by injuries, surgeries, and debilitating diseases. Physical therapy may be effective in people who suffer from chronic pain due to illnesses or other long-term debilitations as well as patients who are injured in accidents. It is estimated that 1 million Americans are treated by physical therapists each day.

Many professional and top college athletes injured on the field often undergo months of physical therapy in order to return to their teams. During the 2008 NFL season, Philadelphia Eagles running back Brian Westbrook was forced to sit out several games with a sprained right ankle. After Westbrook returned, the ankle developed bone spurs, a condition in which extra bone forms as the joint repairs itself. The spurs can be painful because they rub against ligaments and other tissue, so after the season Westbrook had the spurs surgically removed. To rehabilitate his ankle physical therapists designed a program so he would be ready for the 2009 season. Essentially, Westbrook spent the summer dribbling a soccer ball with his right foot. The constant flexing action of the maneuver helped Westbrook improve his flexibility and strength, and soon he was able to perform the activity without pain. "He's in great shape right now. He's worked his tail off. . . . His endurance is phenomenal right now, and he's stronger than an ox,"[29] said Eagles coach Andy Reid.

> " Chiropractors believe the spine helps transmit signals of pain to the rest of the body. "

Statistics show physical therapy is a viable alternative to taking painkillers. In 2009, *Consumer Reports* magazine polled 14,000 patients who suffer from lower back pain; 55 percent of those who were polled said treatment by physical therapists helped ease their pain.

Many patients who seek physical therapy are chronic pain sufferers. Lynn Sygiel, a social worker from Indianapolis, Indiana, suddenly noticed pain and stiffness in her shoulder. The pain was so severe, Sygiel says, that she had trouble sleeping or performing other tasks that had always been simple. "Even pulling up tights was painful," she says. "I had no strength whatsoever."[30] A doctor told her the joint was inflamed due to a hormonal imbalance. The doctor injected her shoulder with an anti-inflammatory drug but told her it would probably take three years before the pain and stiffness eased.

Soon after seeing her doctor, Sygiel started a program of physical therapy. Twice a week the therapist led Sygiel through a series of low-impact exercises designed to improve her shoulder's range of motion. The therapist also applied heat to the shoulder and taught Sygiel stretching exercises to perform at home. Within six weeks Sygiel noticed her pain easing. Six months after starting physical therapy—and well ahead of the doctor's prediction—Sygiel said the pain in her shoulder had eased by some 90 percent.

Chiropractic and Massage Therapy

Chiropractic medicine focuses on relieving pain through manipulation of bones, particularly in the spine. Chiropractors believe the spine helps transmit signals of pain to the rest of the body. Therefore, by manipulating the bones in the spine, the chiropractor seeks to shut down those channels of pain. It is estimated that 30 million people seek treatment from chiropractors each year.

Typically, the chiropractor will spend 15 or 20 minutes per session kneading, twisting, bending, or using other manipulative techniques on the spine, joints, or other bones. "Americans too often choose to pop a pill or seek out elective surgery to treat health problems that could just as effectively—and more safely—be managed by less invasive or non-drug options,"[31] says Donald J. Krippendorf, president of the American Chiropractic Association.

Massachusetts journalist Dana Barbuto suffered from chronic pain in his neck and shoulder for four years. He tried treating the pain with ice, heat, rest, ibuprofen, and physical therapy. Finally, he visited a chiropractor. "Working down my spine, the doctor applied gentle pressure until he found the problem spot," Barbuto said. "Then

> It has long been recognized that marijuana, also known as cannabis, has an analgesic effect.

he pushed a bit more and pop! . . . After the first week, the area was sore, but not painful. . . . I noticed a huge difference in my neck and shoulder area after just two weeks."[32]

Some patients also seek the help of a massage therapist to ease their pain. Unlike chiropractic therapy, which concentrates on bones and joints, massage involves applying pressure to muscles and other soft tissue. "If it helps, if it's very helpful, I encourage my patients that have pursued massage therapy to continue; and I have had many, many people who say that it's very beneficial,"[33] says James Rathmell, a pain specialist at Massachusetts General Hospital.

Medicinal Marijuana

It has long been recognized that marijuana, also known as cannabis, has an analgesic effect. The component of marijuana that gives the drug its narcotic kick—delta-9-tetrahydrocannabinol, or THC—interacts with neurotransmitters, including serotonin, which influence mood. That is what gives most marijuana smokers a dreamy, mellow high. It is also the reason the drug helps block pain.

People who use marijuana for pain usually have chronic pain rather than the acute pain associated with recent injuries. Patients who suffer from chronic pain believe marijuana gives them relief without the side effects of opioids such as Percocet and Vicodin. Among those side effects are depression, allergic reactions, nausea, vomiting, and constipation.

Throughout his life George McMahon sustained numerous broken bones caused by relatively minor accidents. Moreover, after the casts were removed, his body never seemed to heal completely—the pain continued even after the bones had mended. Finally, the Frankton, Texas, man was diagnosed with nail-patella syndrome, a rare genetic disorder that causes brittle bones as well as sore joints and muscle cramps. To treat the pain McMahon relied on a number of prescription painkillers. "I used to gulp pills like a candy addict munching gumdrops,"[34] he says.

> "A lot of pain is regarded as referred pain, meaning an injury or ailment to one part of the body causes pain elsewhere in the body."

Although the pills seemed to reduce his pain, McMahon found himself living in a constant narcotic haze, unable to function.

Frustrated by his inability to live a normal life, McMahon tried marijuana. He says:

> I was to discover that my responses to marijuana were quite different than those of other people. Unlike other individuals who got intoxicated and giggly after smoking marijuana, I simply felt better. I was more alert, my pain was not as debilitating and it was easier for me to move around. The spasms I suffered, particularly in my legs, which prevented me from sleeping eased after smoking marijuana.[35]

McMahon is now an author and advocate for medicinal marijuana. He travels the country speaking about the benefits of the drug while urging state and federal lawmakers to legalize its use as a painkiller. By 2009, through the efforts of McMahon and numerous other advocates for legalization, 14 states had legalized marijuana for medicinal purposes. Others have reduced the penalties for possession of marijuana for medicinal purposes to small fines. However, federal officials have resisted the campaign to legalize marijuana, and in 2005 the U.S. Supreme Court ruled that federal drug agents could arrest medicinal marijuana growers.

Referred Pain

Acupuncture is a technique dating back 5,000 years, first practiced by ancient Chinese physicians. Acupuncturists insert needles into specific parts of the body under the theory that pain can be controlled by interrupting the transmission of energy that flows from point to point. Modern-day physicians concede that there may be some scientific basis to the craft—a lot of pain is regarded as referred pain, meaning an injury or ailment to one part of the body causes pain elsewhere in the body. For example, many patients who have suffered heart attacks know that the first pain they felt from the attack was not in their chests but in their left arms. Likewise, people who eat ice cream too quickly know they can suffer a sudden headache. Both are examples of referred pain.

Therefore, in acupuncture, the practitioner seeks to interrupt the flow of referred pain by inserting needles into the pathways of the pain. According to the National Institutes of Health, more than 2 million Americans a year seek pain relief through acupuncture. One of those patients is Blake Rivas, a 31-year-old Hewlett, New York, woman who suffers from back pain due to a herniated disk, which is an erosion of the spongy material that cushions the bones of the spine. When the spongy disc wears away, bones in the spine come into contact with one another, causing pain. Rivas received injections of painkillers into her back but failed to find much relief until she tried acupuncture. "Sometimes the pain was so bad I was unable to get out of bed," she says. "Since starting acupuncture, I'm back on my feet. I'm wearing high heels again. I feel like a million bucks."[36]

Another alternative therapy that dates back thousands of years is aromatherapy, which may have been first used by Hippocrates in the fifth century B.C. As the name suggests, aromatherapy is the use of scents to cure certain ills. The therapy is based on the theory that scents affect nerve endings. A 2008 study by Ohio State University tested volunteers' reactions to the odors emanating from lemon oil, lavender oil, and distilled water and found little evidence that aromatherapy works. Still, the scientists did not want to discourage people from finding out for themselves. "This is probably the most comprehensive study ever done in this area, but the human body is infinitely complex," said William Malarkey, a professor of internal medicine and one of the authors of the study. "If an individual patient uses these oils and feels better, there's no way we can prove it doesn't improve that person's health."[37]

> " By warming up before their games, athletes can often avoid injuries and the pain they cause. "

A Life Without Pain

Physicians and other health experts believe that the best alternative to using painkilling drugs is to avoid situations that lead to pain. By warming up before their games, athletes can often avoid injuries and the pain they cause. By wearing seatbelts and obeying traffic laws, motorists can avoid accidents that can leave them with painful injuries. By wearing helmets, skateboarders and bicycle riders can avoid painful head injuries.

Meanwhile, medical science is constantly making advances in disease research that may lead to elimination of some of the illnesses that cause chronic pain. A lot of that research focuses on stem cells, which are cells that can be withdrawn from the body and coaxed into becoming cells that can be employed to repair damaged or diseased tissue. At the University of Manchester in Great Britain, scientists are using stem cells withdrawn from bone marrow to repair herniated discs. "This is a really exciting area of research and although it is still early . . . the initial results look very promising,"[38] says Dries Hettinga, a research manager at Back Care, a British foundation that raises money for back pain research.

These developments show how the science of pain management is continually changing, revealing new ways to avoid injuries and cure diseases. In the meantime, accidents are always going to happen, and painful diseases will continue to afflict unfortunate patients. For those people, painkilling drugs are likely to remain an important component of their therapies.

Are There Alternatives to Using Painkillers?

> " Thousands of patients and their doctors have found marijuana to be beneficial in treating the symptoms of AIDS, cancer, multiple sclerosis, glaucoma, and other serious conditions. For many people, marijuana is the only medicine with a suitable degree of safety and efficacy. "

—Marijuana Policy Project, *State by State Medical Marijuana Laws*, 2008. www.mpp.org.

The Marijuana Policy Project is a Washington, D.C.–based organization that advocates liberalization of laws governing the use of marijuana.

> " The campaign to legitimize what is called 'medical' marijuana is based on two propositions: that science views marijuana as medicine, and that DEA [Drug Enforcement Administration] targets sick and dying people using the drug. Neither proposition is true. Smoked marijuana has not withstood the rigors of science—it is not medicine and it is not safe. "

—U.S. Drug Enforcement Administration, "The DEA Position on Marijuana," May 2006. www.usdoj.gov.

The U.S. Drug Enforcement Administration is the chief federal agency responsible for enforcing laws against illegal drug use.

Bracketed quotes indicate conflicting positions.

* Editor's Note: While the definition of a primary source can be narrowly or broadly defined, for the purposes of Compact Research, a primary source consists of: 1) results of original research presented by an organization or researcher; 2) eyewitness accounts of events, personal experience, or work experience; 3) first-person editorials offering pundits' opinions; 4) government officials presenting political plans and/or policies; 5) representatives of organizations presenting testimony or policy.

❝Over the past 30 years, there have been several attempts to have marijuana reclassified to a different schedule which would permit medical use of the drug. All of these attempts have failed. The mere categorization of marijuana as 'medical' by some states fails to carve out any legally recognized exception regarding the drug. Marijuana, in any form, is neither valid nor legal.❞

—California Police Chiefs Association's Task Force on Marijuana Dispensaries, "White Paper on Marijuana Dispensaries," April 22, 2009. www.californiapolicechiefs.org.

The California Police Chiefs Association is the professional association representing the chiefs of municipal police departments in California. The association examines policies, court decisions, and similar issues and provides guidance to its members on how to enforce laws.

❝If a patient is hypnotizable, hypnosis can potentially be a very powerful way to reduce pain at least acutely.❞

—Russell Portenoy, "How Does Hypnosis Work, Can Anyone Be Hypnotized, and When Is It Used?" ABC News, January 2, 2008. http://abcnews.go.com.

Portenoy is chair of the Department of Pain Management, Beth Israel Medical Center, New York.

❝There is a growing body of scientific evidence on the clinical usefulness of hypnosis in pain management. Hypnosis has demonstrated a remarkable versatility in treating a variety of pain syndromes.❞

—Arthur Fass, "Hypnosis for Pain Management," in *Complementary and Integrative Medicine in Pain Management*, ed. Michael I. Weintraub, Ravinder Mamtani, and Marc S. Micozzi. New York: Springer, 2008.

Fass is a cardiologist who practices at Phelps Memorial Hospital in Sleepy Hollow, New York.

❝Proper breathing in a slow, controlled rhythm is the fastest pain reliever you can use. It shifts the mind's attention away from the pain and the body's natural response to pain.❞

—Vijay Vad, *Arthritis Rx*. New York: Gotham, 2006.

Vad is a New York–based physician who specializes in treating arthritis and is the author of the book *Arthritis Rx*.

66 Pain is one of the most distressing of all human conditions; it often taxes the social, emotional, financial, and spiritual abilities of even the most resourceful individuals. 99

—Anne L. Dewar, "Chronic Pain and Mental Illness: A Double Dilemma for All," *Journal of Psychosocial Nursing*, July 2007.

Dewar is an associate professor at the University of British Columbia School of Nursing in Vancouver, Canada.

66 Acupuncture has been around for thousands of years. . . . It was never intended in its origin to be a pain therapy back in ancient China, but it certainly is the most common reason acupuncture is used in this country. 99

—Edward Paul, "Does Acupuncture Relieve Pain, and Can It Be Harmful?" ABC News, January 2, 2008. http://abcnews.go.com.

Paul is an associate professor of family and community medicine at the University of Arizona College of Medicine.

66 Historically, odors have been recognized to have analgesic effects. When Roman soldiers returned from battle, they placed bay leaves in their baths to reduce pain. In ancient Greece, the Corinthian physician, Philonides, recommended pressing cool, scented flowers against the temples to relieve headaches. 99

—Alan R. Hirsch, "Aromatherapy," in *Complementary and Integrative Medicine in Pain Management*, ed. Michael I. Weintraub, Ravinder Mamtani, and Marc S. Micozzi. New York: Springer, 2008.

Hirsch is a physician and director of the Smell and Taste Treatment and Research Foundation of Chicago, Illinois.

Facts and Illustrations

Are There Alternatives to Using Painkillers?

- By 2009, **14 states had legalized marijuana for medicinal use**. Those states include Alaska, California, Colorado, Hawaii, Maine, Maryland, Michigan, Montana, Nevada, New Mexico, Oregon, Rhode Island, Vermont, and Washington.

- According to the *Journal of Family Practice*, **80 percent** of 644 patients suffering from the gastrointestinal ailment irritable bowel syndrome reported a reduction in their pain after undergoing hypnosis.

- A study of 28 AIDS patients conducted by the University of California–San Diego reported **30 percent** reductions in pain among patients who consume medicinal marijuana.

- Studies of the benefits of chiropractic medicine found that in 741 patients who participated in testing, not only was neck and back pain reduced, but many patients reported that their **chiropractic treatments** also eased their migraine headaches.

- The World Health Organization, which is the public health arm of the United Nations, recognizes **30 diseases** and conditions that can be alleviated by acupuncture. One of the conditions on the organization's list is pain.

Massage Can Ease Some Cancer Pain

A study led by the University of Colorado found that massage therapy can help ease the pain of cancer patients. Patients who participated in the study were asked to rate their pain on a scale of 0 to 10, with 0 meaning no pain and 10 meaning the worst pain they could imagine. Patients who received massages said their worst pain dropped by almost 2 points. Members of the control group, who received "simple touch" massage, reported that their pain level dropped by half as much. In simple touch massage, the therapist applies very light pressure to the aching body parts.

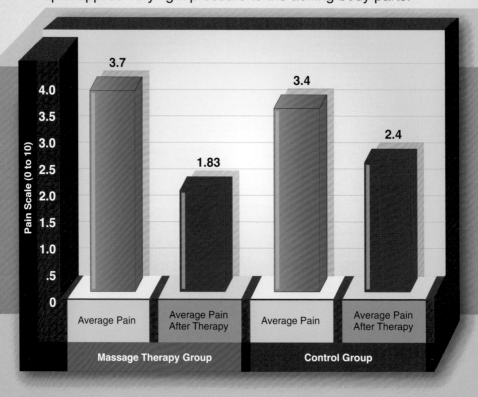

Source: Jean S. Kutner et al., "Massage Therapy Versus Simple Touch to Improve Pain and Mood in Patients with Advanced Cancer," *Annals of Internal Medicine*, September 16, 2008. p. 369.

- In a study published in the *American Pain Society Bulletin*, patients suffering from severe burns reported that their pain eased by **30 to 50 percent** after therapists used techniques to distract them from their pain.

Hypnosis May Cut Postsurgery Pain by More than Half

Women undergoing surgery for breast cancer felt less pain following their procedures if they received hypnotherapy prior to the operations, according to a study led by the Mount Sinai School of Medicine in New York. In the study, patients received 15 minutes of hypnotherapy one hour before their surgeries. Following their surgeries, the patients rated the intensity of their pain at about 22 on a scale of 0 to 100, with 100 being the most unpleasant pain. Members of the control group, who did not receive hypnotherapy before their surgeries, recorded pain intensity scores averaging nearly 48.

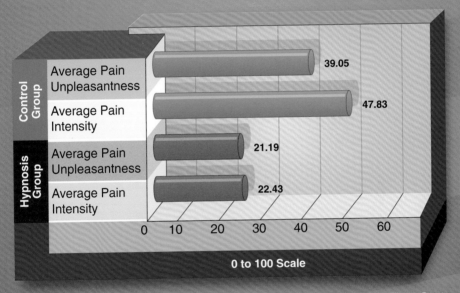

Source: Guy H. Montgomery et al., "A Randomized Clinical Trial of a Brief Hypnosis Intervention to Control Side Effects in Breast Surgery Patients," *Journal of the National Cancer Institute,* September 5, 2007, p. 1,304.

- A comprehensive study of some 40,000 acupuncture patients in Germany revealed that **90 percent** believed their pain subsided after receiving acupuncture treatments, with **50 percent** reporting pain eased within 2 weeks of beginning the therapy.

- A 2008 study by Ohio State University found no evidence to suggest that scents from **lavender oil** or **lemon oil** have any effect on pain.

AIDS Patients Find Relief with Marijuana

A study by San Francisco General Hospital in California found that pain was reduced among AIDS patients who were permitted to smoke marijuana during 5-day stays in the hospital. Before receiving the marijuana, the patients were asked to rate their pain on a scale of 0 to 100, with 100 being the worst pain. Upon entering the hospital, the average pain score among the patients was about 60. About half the patients were given marijuana while half smoked placebo cigarettes. By the end of their stays, the pain among marijuana smokers dropped by about two-thirds while there was little relief reported among the placebo smokers. Seven days after their release, all patients reported pain near their prehospitalization levels.

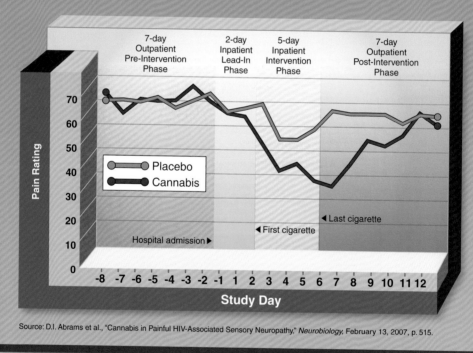

Source: D.I. Abrams et al., "Cannabis in Painful HIV-Associated Sensory Neuropathy," *Neurobiology*, February 13, 2007, p. 515.

- A study conducted on Italian soccer players revealed that knee injuries are reduced by **87 percent** when the athletes warm up on balance boards. Balance boards improve flexibility of joints due to the wobbling motion of their round undersides.

Patients Prefer Chiropractic Care, Acupuncture, and Physical Therapy to Ease Back Pain

Chiropractors, physical therapists, and acupuncturists are not physicians and, therefore, they cannot write prescriptions for painkillers. Nevertheless, 14,000 readers of *Consumer Reports* magazine who responded to a survey said those professionals did more to relieve their low-back pain than family physicians and specialists, who do write prescriptions for painkillers. Nearly 60 percent of the magazine's readers said they were satisfied with the care they received from chiropractors while only about half as many said they were satisfied with the care they received from their family physicians.

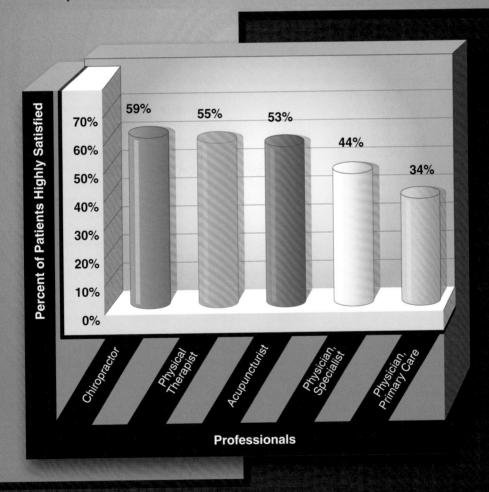

Source: *Consumer Reports*, "Who Helped the Most?" May 2009. www.consumerreports.org.

- A poll commissioned by the American Association of Retired Persons found **72 percent** of respondents in agreement with the statement "Adults should be allowed to legally use marijuana for medical purposes if a physician recommends it."

- Thirty people who participated in a study reported that their lower back pain eased by an average of **28 percent** after exercising 4 days a week over a period of 12 weeks; those who exercised twice a week said their pain eased by an average of **14 percent**.

- According to the *New England Journal of Medicine*, **chiropractic treatments** and **physical therapy** produced no significant improvement in 321 patients treated for lower back pain.

- The *Archives of Internal Medicine* reported a study in which **47 percent** of patients receiving acupuncture said their pain had eased. In contrast, **27 percent** of patients receiving conventional therapy, including painkilling drugs and physical therapy, said their pain had eased.

Key People and Advocacy Groups

Consumer Healthcare Products Association: Based in Washington, D.C., the Consumer Healthcare Products Association is the trade group that represents the manufacturers of nonprescription painkillers as well as other drugs sold over the counter. The association lobbies Congress for laws favorable to the manufacture and sale of nonprescription drugs. The association also commissions scientific studies that explore the effects of nonprescription drugs.

For Grace: The organization works to convince doctors that women in pain are often misdiagnosed and that the pain suffered by women is often much worse than diagnoses would seem to indicate. The Studio City, California, organization was founded by Cynthia Toussaint, a former dance student who spent many years suffering from the painful condition reflex sympathetic dystrophy before a correct diagnosis was finally rendered.

David Graham: The scientist for the U.S. Food and Drug Administration recognized the dangers of Vioxx, but his warnings were ignored. Instead, Graham brought his concerns to Congress, which helped put pressure on the drug's manufacturer, Merck, to withdraw the prescription painkiller from the market. Merck has since agreed to pay $5 billion in damages to some 44,000 patients or their families who suffered heart attacks and strokes after taking Vioxx.

Felix Hoffman: The father of German chemist Felix Hoffman suffered from arthritis but was unable to take salicylic acid because it troubled his stomach. Hoffman buffered the drug by adding salt and the chemical acetyl chloride to create acetylsalicylic acid, making it more friendly to stomachs. The drug company where Hoffman worked, Bayer, named his creation aspirin.

National Consumers League: The organization has taken positions on many issues that affect Americans, including the overuse of nonprescription drugs, and lobbies Congress for more effective laws that protect consumers. A survey conducted by the Washington, D.C., group found that 44 percent of people who consume nonprescription painkillers exceed the recommended maximum doses that are listed on the drugs' labels.

National Organization for the Reform of Marijuana Laws: The Washington, D.C.–based group lobbies lawmakers to support liberalization of the laws that govern marijuana use in America. The group has compiled numerous studies showing the benefits of marijuana as a painkiller and has also commissioned surveys reflecting strong public support for legalization of medicinal marijuana.

Public Citizen: Public Citizen is a consumer rights group that advocates for laws that protect consumers from dangerous drugs. The group has sued the U.S. Food and Drug Administration in an effort to have some prescription painkillers withdrawn from the market. Also, Public Citizen has long advocated for stricter warning labels to be placed on nonprescription painkillers.

Angel Raich and Diane Monson: Diane Monson, who grew marijuana for medicinal purposes, and Angel Raich, who used marijuana as an analgesic, sued the U.S. Justice Department to prevent federal agents from arresting growers of medicinal marijuana. The case was heard by the U.S. Supreme Court in 2005, which ruled that federal agents can pursue prosecutions against medicinal marijuana growers. However, the court also ruled that states have the right to legalize marijuana for medicinal purposes, and by 2009, 14 states had passed laws legalizing medical marijuana.

Friedrich Sertürner: In 1804 the German pharmacist Friedrich Sertürner extracted a painkilling drug from opium. He called it morphine after Morpheus, the Greek god of dreams. Soon morphine would be employed by doctors to treat battlefield wounds suffered by soldiers. Today morphine and other opiate-based painkillers are prescribed for cancer patients and others whose pain is severe.

Chronology

Fifth century B.C.
Greek physician Hippocrates urges his patients to chew willow bark for pain relief; later, chemists will determine the bark contains a key ingredient of aspirin.

1804
German pharmacist Friedrich Sertürner extracts the painkilling drug morphine from opium.

1893
German chemist Felix Hoffman buffers salicylic acid, making it digestible. The new drug is named aspirin by Hoffman's employer, drug maker Bayer.

1988
Doctors discover two forms of cyclooxygenase in the body: Cox-1 and Cox-2. The discovery leads to the development of the painkilling Cox-2 inhibitors Vioxx, Celebrex, and Bextra.

1800

1900

1990

1799
English chemist Humphry Davy discovers the calming qualities of nitrous oxide.

1906
Congress passes the U.S. Pure Food and Drug Act, giving the federal government power over the regulation of painkillers and other prescription drugs. Later, Congress creates the U.S. Food and Drug Administration (FDA) to regulate drugs.

1842
Ether vapors are first employed as a general anesthesia for surgery patients.

1955
Acetaminophen goes into widespread use as a painkiller when Tylenol is introduced to the market.

1845
Horace Wells becomes the first dentist to sedate a patient using nitrous oxide.

1969
British doctors prescribe ibuprofen as a painkiller for arthritis patients.

1992
Congress passes the U.S. Prescription Drug User Fee Act, requiring drug companies to pay fees to have their products assessed for safety by the FDA.

2002
Drug agents seize marijuana plants from the home of Diane Monson, who claimed to grow the plants for medicinal purposes; three years later the U.S. Supreme Court ruled that the federal government has the right to prosecute growers of medicinal marijuana.

2000
Concerns about Vioxx start surfacing, indicating the drug could double the chances of causing heart attack and stroke.

2005
The FDA orders Bextra withdrawn from the market; Celebrex is permitted to stay on the market, but the drug must carry a black box warning.

1990   **2000**   **2010**

1996
OxyContin goes on the market in America; the delayed-action narcotic painkiller marks a step forward in managing pain but is soon widely abused by drug users.

2004
Merck, the manufacturer of Vioxx, withdraws the drug from the market.

2007
Merck agrees to pay nearly $5 billion in damages to some 44,000 patients who suffered heart attacks and strokes while taking Vioxx.

1999
Vioxx is approved by the FDA.

2008
Pfizer, the distributor of Bextra and Celebrex, agrees to pay $900 million to some 8,000 patients who suffered heart attacks and strokes while taking the drugs.

2009
An FDA advisory panel recommends cutting the maximum dosages for acetaminophen products due to concerns that the drug causes liver damage.

Related Organizations

American Chronic Pain Association

PO Box 850

Rocklin, CA 95677

phone: (800) 533-3231 • fax: (916) 632-3208

e-mail: acpa@pacbell.net • Web site: www.theacpa.org

The American Chronic Pain Association organizes support groups for sufferers of chronic pain and also provides advice to members on how to find doctors and therapists and how to choose painkilling drugs. Visitors to the organization's Web site can download copies of the *American Chronic Pain Association Chronicle*, a quarterly newsletter that provides news about advances in pain management.

American Medical Association

515 N. State St.

Chicago, IL 60610

phone: (800) 621-8335

Web site: www.ama-assn.org

The national association representing American physicians has provided its members with direction for treating pain and prescribing painkilling drugs. In 2009 the organization's Council on Scientific Affairs declared that despite tremendous advances in pain management and the development of new painkilling drugs, doctors do not provide many of their patients adequate pain relief.

American Society of Anesthesiologists

520 N. Northwest Hwy.

Park Ridge, IL 60068-2573

phone: (847) 825-5586 • fax: (847) 825-1692

e-mail: mail@asahq.org • Web site: www.asahq.org

The society is the professional association of physicians who administer anesthesia to patients who undergo major surgeries. By following the link to "Patient Education," students can find many resources on anesthesia and drugs that are typically employed. Also, students can view the video *Pain Medicine*, in which leading anesthesiologists discuss pain medicines, their proper use, and the myths surrounding their use.

International Association for the Study of Pain (IASP)

111 Queen Anne Ave. North, Suite 501

Seattle, WA 98109-4955

phone: (206) 283-0311 • fax: (206) 283-9403

e-mail: iaspdesk@iasp-pain.org • Web site www.iasp-pain.org

The IASP is composed of physicians who treat pain. The organization pursues scientific research into pain and provides education to its members on the latest advancements in pain management. Visitors to the organization's Web site can review the definitions of pain and related topics that the organization has established.

Marijuana Policy Project

PO Box 77492

Washington, DC 20013

phone: (202) 462-5747

e-mail: info@mpp.org • Web site: www.mpp.org

The Marijuana Policy Project coordinates efforts to liberalize marijuana laws in America, particularly laws regulating the use of medicinal marijuana. Visitors to the organization's Web site can download the 2008 report, *State by State Medical Marijuana Laws*, which provides readers with the status of efforts in all 50 states to legalize medicinal marijuana.

Substance Abuse and Mental Health Services Administration (SAMHSA)

1 Choke Cherry Rd., Room 8-1054

Rockville, MD 20857

phone: (240) 276-2000

Web site: www.samhsa.gov

An agency of the U.S. Health and Human Services Department, SAMHSA studies drug use and helps develop programs for drug abusers. Visitors to SAMHSA's Web site can download the 2009 report *Trends in Nonmedical Use of Prescription Painkillers: 2002 to 2007.*

Tufts Center for the Study of Drug Development

Tufts University

75 Kneeland St., Suite 1100

Boston, MA 02111

phone: (617) 636-2170 • fax: (617) 636-2425

e-mail: csdd@tufts.edu • Web site: http://csdd.tufts.edu

The Tufts Center for the Study of Drug Development charts trends that guide the development of new prescription drugs, including painkillers. The center studies factors such as the money drug companies invest in new drugs, the length of time drugs must spend in clinical trials, and the influence of the U.S. Food and Drug Administration on the approval process. Visitors to the organization's Web site can download copies of *Outlook*, the center's annual report detailing trends in the American prescription drug industry.

U.S. Drug Enforcement Administration (DEA)

2401 Jefferson Davis Hwy.

Alexandria, VA 22301

phone: (202) 307-1000

Web site: www.usdoj.gov/dea

The DEA enforces federal laws that prohibit the trafficking of illegal drugs, including marijuana sold for medicinal purposes and opiate-based painkillers sold on the black market. The agency also assists state and local police departments in their investigations of drug traffickers. Fact sheets on OxyContin and other opiate-based painkillers can be found on the DEA's Web site.

U.S. Food and Drug Administration (FDA)

5600 Fishers Ln.

Rockville, MD 20857-0001

phone: (888) 463-6332

Web site: www.fda.gov

All nonprescription and prescription drugs sold in the United States must be approved by the FDA. In assessing painkillers and other drugs, the agency's staff of biologists, chemists, and other scientists reviews the results of clinical trials submitted by drug companies. Students can find many resources about painkillers, clinical trials, and other issues involving the regulation of painkillers on the FDA's Web site.

White House Office of National Drug Control Policy

PO Box 6000

Rockville, MD 20849-6000

phone: (800) 666-3332

Web site: www.whitehousedrugpolicy.gov

The White House Office of National Drug Control Policy develops national strategies for combating drug abuse and coordinates the activities of several federal agencies charged with overseeing scientific research on drugs, enforcement of drug laws, and other areas that cover drug use and abuse. The 2008 report *Prescription for Danger: A Report on the Troubling Trend of Prescription and Over-the-Counter Drug Abuse Among the Nation's Teens* can be downloaded at the agency's Web site.

For Further Research

Books

Jerome Bettis, *The Bus: My Life In and Out of a Helmet*. New York: Doubleday, 2007.

Richard Glen Boire and Kevin Feeney, *Medical Marijuana Law*. Oakland, CA: Ronin, 2007.

Wendy Chapkis and Richard Webb, *Dying to Get High: Marijuana as Medicine*. New York: New York University Press, 2008.

Robert S. Kunkel, *Headaches: A Cleveland Clinic Handbook*. Cleveland, OH: Cleveland Clinic, 2007.

Tony Mandarich, *My Dirty Little Secrets—Steroids, Alcohol and God: The Tony Mandarich Story*. Ann Arbor, MI: Modern History, 2009.

Tom Nesi, *Poison Pills: The Untold Story of the Vioxx Drug Scandal*. New York: Thomas Dunne, 2008.

Vijay Vad, *Arthritis Rx*. New York: Gotham, 2006.

Periodicals

Marshall Allen and Alex Richards, "The Painful Truth About Nevada," *Las Vegas Sun*, July 6, 2008.

Marcia Angell, "Charting a New Course at the FDA," *Boston Globe*, April 6, 2009.

Linda Bren, "Managing Migraines," *FDA Consumer*, March/April 2006.

David Graham, "Pain Management," *Toronto Star*, October 11, 2007.

Gardiner Harris, "Ban Is Advised on 2 Top Pills for Pain Relief," *New York Times*, July 1, 2009.

———, "House Passes Bill Giving More Power to the FDA," *New York Times*, September 20, 2007.

Dick Heller, "No-Hitter in '91 Left Ryan in Seventh Heaven," *Washington Times*, May 8, 2006.

Dana Jennings, "Post-Op Strategies: Painkillers, to Start," *New York Times*, January 27, 2009.

Mike Jensen, "Tackling the Pain," *Philadelphia Inquirer*, June 7, 2009.

Victoria McEvoy, "A Doctor's Dilemma: Prescribing Pain Pills Is Getting Trickier," *Boston Globe*, February 4, 2008.

Alan Mozes, "FDA Seeks Better Regulation of Painkillers," *U.S. News & World Report*, February 9, 2009.

Tara Parker-Pope, "Herbs, Hypnosis May Ease Common Bowel Pain," *New York Times*, February 18, 2008.

Dennis Romboy, "Painkillers, the Dark Side of Sports," *Salt Lake City Deseret Morning News*, October 27, 2007.

Karl Stark, "Merck Offers Billions for Vioxx Claims; The Deal, Worth up to $4.85 Billion, Would Settle 26,000 Suits over the Discontinued Pain Reliever," *Philadelphia Inquirer*, November 10, 2007.

Internet Sources

"Gonzalez, Attorney General, et al. v. Raich et al.," opinion of the U.S. Supreme Court in the medicinal marijuana case, FindLaw, June 6, 2005. http://caselaw.lp.findlaw.com/scripts/getcase.pl?court=US&vol=000&invol=03-1454.

International Association for the Study of Pain, "Pain Terminology," November 29, 2007. www.iasp-pain.org/AM/Template.cfm?Section=Pain_Definitions&Template=/CM/HTMLDisplay.cfm&ContentID=1728.

Mayo Clinic, "How You Feel Pain," February 13, 2009. www.mayoclinic.com/health/pain/PN00017.

National Headache Foundation, "Migraine," 2009. www.headaches.org/education/Headache_Topic_Sheets/Migraine.

National Library of Medicine, "Pain," July 12, 2009. www.nlm.nih.gov/medlineplus/pain.html.

Source Notes

Overview

1. Quoted in Debra Gordon, "The Painful Truth," *Consumer Digest,* September/October 2005. www.debra gordon.com.
2. Quoted in Dick Heller, "No-Hitter in '91 Left Ryan in Seventh Heaven," *Washington Times,* May 8, 2006, p. C-10.
3. Jeff Jay and Jerry A. Boriskin, *At Wit's End: What You Need to Know When a Loved One Is Diagnosed with Addiction and Mental Illness.* Center City, MN: Hazelden, 2007, pp. 203–4.
4. Quoted in Peter McQuaid, "Paula Abdul, Straight Up," *Ladies Home Journal,* June 2009. www.lhj.com.
5. Quoted in Gardiner Harris, "Ban Is Advised on 2 Top Pills for Pain Relief," *New York Times,* July 1, 2009, p. A-1.

How Do Painkillers Affect the Body?

6. Quoted in Paul Doyle, "Pain Killers: Neither Breaks Nor Sprains Will Keep Some Athletes Off the Playing Field," *Hartford (CT) Courant,* November 19, 2002, p. C-1.
7. International Association for the Study of Pain, "Pain Terminology," November 29, 2007. www.iasp-pain. org.
8. Quoted in Stanford School of Medicine, "Physical Pain Aggravates Majority of Americans, According to Poll from Stanford, ABC News and *USA Today,*" news release, May 9, 2005. http://med.stanford.edu.
9. Quoted in Claudia Kalb, Karen Springen, Joan Raymond, and Anne Underwood, "Taking a New Look at Pain," *Newsweek,* May 19, 2003, p. 44.

10. Darin Workman, *The Percussionists' Guide to Injury Treatment and Prevention.* New York: Routledge, 2006, p. 14.
11. Drew Pinsky, *When Painkillers Become Dangerous.* Center City, MN: Hazelden, 2004, p. 4.
12. Quoted in Linda Bren, "Managing Migraines," *FDA Consumer,* March/April 2006, p. 31.

What Are the Dangers of Painkillers?

13. Quoted in Mike Jensen, "Tackling the Pain," *Philadelphia Inquirer,* June 7, 2009, p. E-11.
14. Quoted in Jensen, "Tackling the Pain," p. E-10.
15. White House Office of National Drug Control Policy, *Prescription for Danger: A Report on the Troubling Trend of Prescription and Over-the-Counter Drug Abuse Among the Nation's Teens,* January 2008. www.theantidrug.com.
16. Tom Woerner, "Pharmacy Robbers Steal Only Prescription Drugs," *Dunn (NC) Daily Record,* July 10, 2009. www.mydailyrecord.com.
17. Quoted in National Consumers League, "New Survey Reveals Uninformed Consumers Taking Dangerous Risks with OTC Painkillers," news release, January 30, 2003. www.nclnet. org.
18. Quoted in Associated Press, "Teens Suffering from Rebound Headaches," *USA Today,* June 14, 2004. www.usa today.com.
19. Quoted in Medical News Today, "Children Overdoing OTC Painkillers," July 18, 2004. www.medical newstoday.com.
20. Quoted in Emily Sohn, "Not Just

a Headache," *Health*, May 2004, p. 146.

21. Quoted in Sohn, "Not Just a Headache," p. 147.

22. Quoted in Jensen, "Tackling the Pain," p. E-10.

How Effective Is Government Oversight of Painkillers?

23. Quoted in Saundra Young, "FDA Requires New Labels for Over-the-Counter Painkillers," CNN, April 28, 2009. www.cnn.com.

24. Quoted in Chris Mondics, "FDA Safety Called Lacking," *Albany (NY) Times Union*, November 19, 2004, p. A-1.

25. Quoted in Diedtra Henderson, "Calls Are Mounting for Revamp of FDA," *Boston Globe*, December 25, 2004, p. B-5.

26. Marcia Angell, "Charting a New Course for the FDA," *Boston Globe*, April 6, 2009. www.boston.com.

27. Marcia Angell, "Taking Back the FDA," *Boston Globe*, February 26, 2007. www.boston.com.

Are There Alternatives to Using Painkillers?

28. Quoted in Benedict Carey, "Harnessing the Power of the Mind," *Lancaster (PA) Intelligencer Journal*, January 25, 2004, p. 1.

29. Quoted in Andre Williams, "Westbrook Springs, Dribbles Soccer Ball,"

Allentown (PA) Morning Call, July 29, 2009. http://blogs.mcall.com.

30. Quoted in Patricia Hagen, "Thawing Out Frozen Shoulder," *Saturday Evening Post*, September/October 2008, p. 62.

31. Quoted in *Medical News*, "Survey Shows Need for Conservative, Drug-Free Options," November 20, 2004. www.news-medical.net.

32. Dana Barbuto, "Spine-Tingling Facts: Manipulating the Pain Away," *Quincy (MA) Patriot Ledger*, March 29, 2006, p. 14.

33. James Rathmell, "Massage Feels Good When It's Being Done. Can It Provide Continued Pain Relief?" ABC News, January 2, 2008. http://abcnews.go.com.

34. George McMahon and Christopher Largen, *Prescription Pot: A Leading Advocate's Heroic Battle to Legalize Medical Marijuana.* Far Hills, NJ: New Horizon, 2003, p. 47.

35. McMahon and Largen, *Prescription Pot*, p. 48.

36. Quoted in Debbie Geiger, "Easing Back Pain the Alternative Way," *Newsday*, February 6, 2007, p. B-8.

37. Quoted in *Medical News*, "Aromatherapy and Pain Relief?" March 4, 2008. www.news-medical.net.

38. Quoted in BBC News, "Stem Cell Cure Hope for Back Pain," November 30, 2006. http://news.bbc.co.uk.

List of Illustrations

How Do Painkillers Affect the Body?

What Are the Dangers of Painkillers?

How Effective Is Government Oversight of Painkillers?

Are There Alternatives to Using Painkillers?

Index

About the Author

Hal Marcovitz, a writer based in Chalfont, Pennsylvania, has written more than 130 books for young readers. His other titles in the Compact Research series include *Religious Fundamentalism*, *Bipolar Disorders*, *Phobias*, *Hepatitis*, and *Meningitis*.